SpringerBriefs in Statistics

SpringerBriefs present concise summaries of cutting-edge research and practical applications across a wide spectrum of fields. Featuring compact volumes of 50 to 125 pages, the series covers a range of content from professional to academic. Typical topics might include:

- A timely report of state-of-the art analytical techniques
- A bridge between new research results, as published in journal articles, and a contextual literature review
- A snapshot of a hot or emerging topic
- An in-depth case study or clinical example
- A presentation of core concepts that students must understand in order to make independent contributions

SpringerBriefs in Statistics showcase emerging theory, empirical research, and practical application in Statistics from a global author community.

SpringerBriefs are characterized by fast, global electronic dissemination, standard publishing contracts, standardized manuscript preparation and formatting guidelines, and expedited production schedules.

More information about this series at http://www.springer.com/series/8921

Ingwer Borg · Patrick J. F. Groenen
Patrick Mair

Applied Multidimensional Scaling and Unfolding

Second Edition

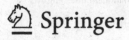

Ingwer Borg
Westfälische Wilhelms-Universität
Münster
Germany

Patrick J. F. Groenen
Econometric Institute
Erasmus University Rotterdam
Rotterdam
The Netherlands

Patrick Mair
Department of Psychology
Harvard University
Cambridge, MA
USA

Additional material to this book can be downloaded from http://extras.springer.com.

ISSN 2191-544X   ISSN 2191-5458 (electronic)
SpringerBriefs in Statistics
ISBN 978-3-319-73470-5   ISBN 978-3-319-73471-2 (eBook)
https://doi.org/10.1007/978-3-319-73471-2

Library of Congress Control Number: 2018934861

Mathematics Subject Classification (2010): 91C15

Printed on acid-free paper

This Springer imprint is published by the registered company Springer International Publishing AG
part of Springer Nature
The registered company address is: Gewerbestrasse 11, 6330 Cham, Switzerland

Preface

Multidimensional scaling (MDS) is a powerful statistical method that maps proximity data on pairs of objects (i.e., data expressing the similarity or the dissimilarity of pairs of objects) into distances between points in a multidimensional space. The space is usually two-dimensional, sometimes also three-dimensional, and seldom more than three-dimensional. Unfolding is a related method for preference data (e.g., persons' ratings on choice objects such as consumer goods). It maps these data into distances between points representing the persons and points representing the choice objects.

The purpose of MDS and unfolding is often just visualizing the data so it becomes easier for the user to explore and to understand their structure. However, both MDS and unfolding can also be used to test a variety of structural hypotheses about the data or even psychological theories of judgment or choice. Thousands of publications have used MDS and unfolding in these ways.

This book is a brief introduction to MDS and unfolding. It discusses the issues that always come up when MDS or unfolding is used in substantive research, and it shows how to actually run such analyses. The aim is conceptual understanding and practical know-how rather than mathematical precision and proof. It is more like a driving lesson, not like engineering a car. These are different things, and the engineer is not necessarily a better driver.

In this second edition, we focus much more on R packages and the R environment than we did in the first edition. However, we decided not to drop other computer packages (such as SPSS and its modules, in particular), because many users are (still?) using these programs. Moreover, some of these programs have features that are not available in R yet. On the other hand, we mention highly special stand-alone programs only occasionally, since many of them are hard to get and difficult to use.

This edition also puts much more emphasis on unfolding. Unfolding was almost completely neglected in the first edition, since nobody used it, even though it is a powerful method and an interesting model. Things have changed recently: Unfolding seems to become more popular in substantive research and in consulting.

With regard to MDS, we introduce and explain recent developments that are concerned with the goodness of an MDS solution and with its substantive interpretation. They are particularly important for the MDS user, for reviewers, and for journal editors. For example, MDS users can now test the statistical significance of MDS (and unfolding) solutions using methods that require computer simulations that were difficult to run within traditional statistics packages but that are now easily feasible within the R environment.

We also present various new examples of how to run an MDS or an unfolding job using R. These examples are almost all substantively relevant and not just contrived illustrative examples. Most data that we use in this book are also readily available in the R package SMACOF so that the user can check our analyses.

To make our cases as concrete as possible, we repeatedly show R scripts for running the jobs. In these scripts, we tried adhering to the R etiquette of writing R code, but did not follow it strictly where it would waste too much space. For example, we often use the semicolon to write more than just one command per line. Prettier code can easily be generated by marking the code and then typing Ctrl +Shift+A in RStudio, for example, or by using the `tidy_source()` function in the formatR package. The scripts shown in this book (and a few additional ones) are also available, in prettier form, in the supplementary script file. Additional material to this book can be downloaded from http://extras.springer.com. It should also be noted that some plots do not correspond exactly to those produced by the various scripts. Rather, some plots were slightly edited by hand to unclutter, in particular, the labels attached to the points in scatter plots.

Münster, Germany   Ingwer Borg
Rotterdam, The Netherlands   Patrick J. F. Groenen
Cambridge, USA   Patrick Mair

Contents

1 First Steps 1
   1.1   Basic Ideas of Multidimensional Scaling 1
   1.2   Basic Ideas of Unfolding 8
   1.3   Summary 10
   References 10

2 The Purpose of MDS and Unfolding 11
   2.1   MDS for Visualizing Proximity Data 11
   2.2   MDS for Uncovering Latent Dimensions of Judgment 13
   2.3   Distance Formulas as Models of Judgment 16
   2.4   MDS for Testing Structural Hypotheses 19
   2.5   Unfolding as a Psychological Model of Preference 23
   2.6   Summary 27
   References 27

3 The Fit of MDS and Unfolding Solutions 29
   3.1   The Global Stress of MDS Solutions 29
   3.2   Evaluating Stress Statistically 33
   3.3   Stress and MDS Dimensionality 35
   3.4   Stress Per Point 36
   3.5   Conditions Causing High Stress in MDS 38
   3.6   Stress in Unfolding 39
   3.7   Stability of MDS Solutions 39
   3.8   Summary 41
   References 41

4 Proximities 43
   4.1   Direct Proximities 43
   4.2   Derived Proximities 45
   4.3   Proximities from Index Conversions 46

4.4   Co-occurrence Data.................................   47
4.5   The Gravity Model for Co-occurrences   49
4.6   Summary   51
References   51

5   Variants of MDS Models   53
5.1   The Type of Regression in MDS.....................   53
5.2   Euclidean and Other Distances   57
5.3   MDS of Asymmetric Proximities.....................   57
5.4   Modeling Individual Differences in MDS.............   60
5.5   Scaling Replicated Proximities......................   63
5.6   Weighting Proximities in MDS   64
5.7   Summary   65
References   65

6   Confirmatory MDS   67
6.1   Weak Confirmatory MDS   67
6.2   External Side Constraints on the Dimensions   68
6.3   Regional Axial Restrictions   70
6.4   Circular and Spherical MDS   72
6.5   Challenges of Confirmatory MDS   74
6.6   Summary   75
References   75

7   Typical Mistakes in MDS   77
7.1   Assigning the Wrong Polarity to Proximities   77
7.2   Using Too Few Iterations   77
7.3   Using the Wrong Initial Configuration   78
7.4   Doing Nothing to Avoid Suboptimal Local Minima   81
7.5   Not Recognizing Degenerate Solutions................   81
7.6   Meaningless Comparisons of Different MDS Solutions   84
7.7   Evaluating Stress Blindly   85
7.8   Always Interpreting Principal Axes Dimensions   86
7.9   Always Interpreting Dimensions or Directions   89
7.10   Poorly Dealing with Disturbing Points   91
7.11   Scaling Almost-Equal Proximities   92
7.12   Summary   92
References   93

8   Unfolding   95
8.1   Unfolding in Three-Dimensional Space   95
8.2   Multidimensional Versus Multiple Unfolding   98
8.3   Conditionalities in Unfolding........................   99
8.4   Stability of Unfolding Solutions......................   100

	8.5	Degenerate Unfolding Solutions	100
	8.6	Special Unfolding Models	101
	8.7	Summary	103
	References		104
9	**MDS Algorithms**		105
	9.1	Classical MDS	105
	9.2	Iterative MDS Algorithms	107
	9.3	Summary	109
	References		110
10	**MDS Software**		111
	10.1	Proxscal	111
	10.2	The R Package smacof	115
		10.2.1 Functions in smacof	116
		10.2.2 A Simple MDS Example	118
	References		120
Index			121

Chapter 1
First Steps

Abstract The basic ideas of MDS are introduced doing MDS by hand. Then, MDS is done using statistical software. The goodness of the MDS configuration is evaluated by correlating its distances with the data. Unfolding is introduced with a small example.

Keywords MDS · Iteration · Proximities · Dimensional interpretation
Goodness of fit · Unfolding

1.1 Basic Ideas of Multidimensional Scaling

The basic ideas of MDS are easily explained using a small example. Consider Table 1.1. It contains the correlations of different crimes in 50 US states. The correlations show, for example, that if there are many cases of Assault in a state, then there are also many cases of Murder ($r = 0.81$). We now scale these correlations via MDS. This means that we try to represent the seven crimes by seven points in a geometric space so that any two points lie the *closer* together the *greater* the correlation of the crimes that these points represent.

To reach this goal, we take seven cards, and write the name of one crime on each of them, from Murder to Auto Theft. These cards are then placed on a table in an arbitrary arrangement (Fig. 1.1). Their distances are measured (Fig. 1.2) and compared with the correlations in Table 1.1. This comparison shows that the configuration in Fig. 1.1 does not represent the data in the desired sense. For example, the cards for Murder and Assault should be relatively close together, because these crimes are correlated with 0.81, whereas the cards for Murder and Larceny should be farther apart, as these crimes are correlated with only 0.06. We, therefore, try to move the cards repeatedly in small steps ("iteratively") so that the distances correspond more closely to the data. Figure 1.3 demonstrates in which directions the cards should be shifted to improve the correspondence of data and distances.

Improving a given configuration iteratively by hand can be fairly tedious. It also does not guarantee convergence to a stable and optimal configuration. So, let an

© The Author(s) 2018

I. Borg et al., *Applied Multidimensional Scaling and Unfolding*,
SpringerBriefs in Statistics, https://doi.org/10.1007/978-3-319-73471-2_1

Table 1.1: Correlations of crime rates in 50 US states

Crime	Murder	Rape	Robbery	Assault	Burglary	Larceny	Auto Theft
Murder	1.00	0.52	0.34	0.81	0.28	0.06	0.11
Rape	0.52	1.00	0.55	0.70	0.68	0.60	0.44
Robbery	0.34	0.55	1.00	0.56	0.62	0.44	0.62
Assault	0.81	0.70	0.56	1.00	0.52	0.32	0.33
Burglary	0.28	0.68	0.62	0.52	1.00	0.80	0.70
Larceny	0.06	0.60	0.44	0.32	0.80	1.00	0.55
Auto Theft	0.11	0.44	0.62	0.33	0.70	0.55	1.00

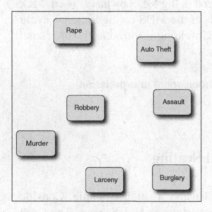

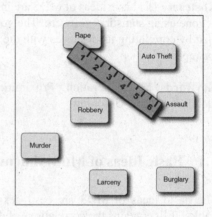

Fig. 1.1: Initial configuration for an MDS of the data in Table 1.1

Fig. 1.2: Measuring distances with a ruler

MDS computer algorithm do the job. It systematically moves the points step by step to improve the fit to the data.

There exist many good MDS programs. One such program is PROXSCAL, a module of SPSS. To use PROXSCAL, we first save the correlation matrix of Table 1.1 in a file that we call 'CorrCrimes.sav'. Then, we only need some clicks in PROXSCAL's menus (click: Analyze > Scale > Multidimensional Scaling (PROXSCAL)) or, alternatively, execute the following commands:

```
1  GET FILE='CorrCrimes.sav'.
2  PROXSCAL VARIABLES=Murder to AutoTheft
3      /TRANSFORMATION=INTERVAL
4      /PROXIMITIES=SIMILARITIES .
```

The PROXIMITIES sub-command informs the program that the data—called *proximities* in this context, a generic term for both *similarity* and *dissimilarity* data—must be interpreted as similarities by the program. That is, small data values should be mapped

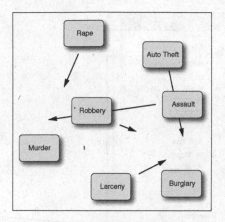

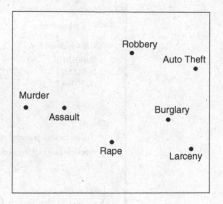

Fig. 1.3: Directions for point movements to improve the MDS configuration

Fig. 1.4: Optimal computer-generated MDS solution

into large distances, and large data values into small distances. Also, we want to map the correlations linearly into MDS distances, preserving their differences ("intervals") in the distances. In PROXSCAL, we thus request /TRANSFORMATION=INTERVAL. No further specifications are needed. The program uses its default settings to generate an MDS solution (Fig. 1.4).

Many other programs exist for MDS. One example is the MDS module in SYSTAT. SYSTAT can be run using commands, or by clicking on various options in a graphical user interface. Having loaded the correlation matrix as our data, we call the MDS module and its menu in Fig. 1.5. We select the variables Murder, Rape, etc., and leave all other specifications as they are, except the one for "Regression", where we request that the MDS program should optimize the relation of data to distances in the sense of a least-squares *linear* regression. Clicking on the OK button makes the program find and plot an MDS configuration.

A third implementation is the mds() function of the R (R Core Team 2017) package SMACOF (De Leeuw and Mair 2009). SMACOF is open source and, most importantly, allows using the sheer boundless capabilities of the R environment and its thousands of software packages for additional analyses, simulations, and graphics. So, we will mostly use SMACOF in this book.

SMACOF is run by commands. A few commands suffice to do the MDS analysis of the given data. Note that SMACOF always requires that the data either come as dissimilarities, or that they have been converted to dissimilarities (accomplished here by the sim2diss function).

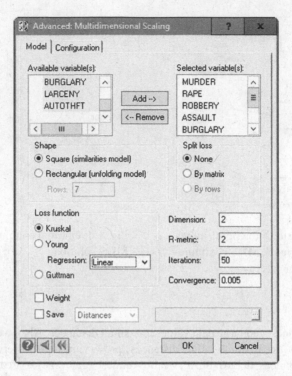

Fig. 1.5: GUI of the MDS module in SYSTAT

```
1  library(smacof)  ## load smacof package
2  data(crimes) ## load data set "crimes"
3  diss <- sim2diss(crimes, method="corr")   ## correlations-->dissimilarities
4  result <- mds(diss, type="interval")   ## run MDS and store in "result"
5  result  ## show basic information about the MDS job
6  names(result)  ## show names of what is contained in object "result"
7  plot(result)  ## plot MDS configuration (as in Fig. 1.6)
```

Figure 1.6 shows these commands in the upper left-hand panel of RSTUDIO, a graphical user interface for R. If you run these commands, an MDS solution is generated and stored in an object called "result" (along with other information about the MDS job; see p. 119). The MDS configuration is plotted in the lower right-hand panel of RSTUDIO.

All three computer programs—PROXSCAL, SYSTAT, and SMACOF—generate essentially the same MDS solution for the crime data. This solution is not only optimal, but also quite good, as Fig. 1.7 shows. This scatter plot demonstrates that our data and the corresponding MDS distances have an almost perfect linear relation ($r = -0.989$). Hence, the data are properly *visualized* and the MDS distances have a clear meaning: The closer two points in the MDS solution, the higher the correlation of the variables that they represent.

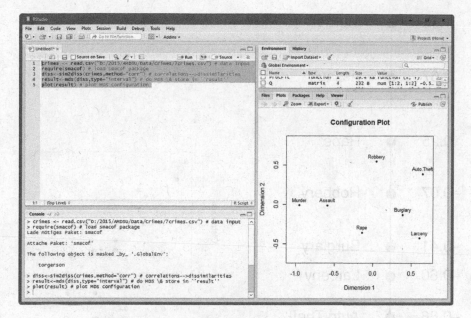

Fig. 1.6: Running an MDS for the crime data using SMACOF out of RSTUDIO

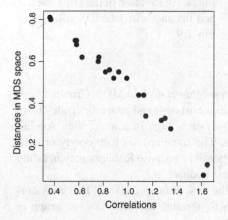

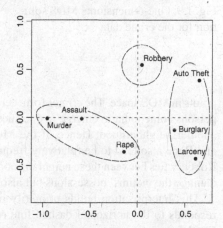

Fig. 1.7: Relation of data in Table 1.1
and distances in Fig. 1.4

Fig. 1.8: MDS solution with two interpretations: neighborhoods and principal axes (crossed lines)

What has been gained by analyzing the crime data via MDS? First, instead of 21
correlations, we get a simple picture of the empirical interrelations. This allows us
to actually *see* and more easily explore the structure of the correlations: The higher
the correlation of two crimes, the smaller the distance between the corresponding

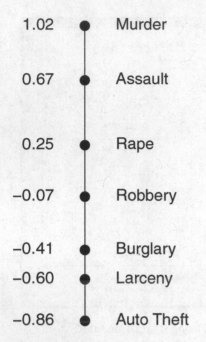

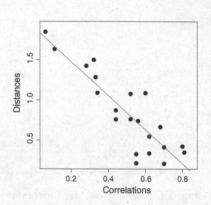

Fig. 1.9: One-dimensional MDS solution for the crime data

Fig. 1.10: Relation of data in Table 1.1
and distances in 1d MDS solution in
Fig. 1.9

points in MDS space. The crimes form certain *neighborhoods* in MDS: Crimes where
persons come to harm emerge in one such neighborhood, and property crimes form
another neighborhood. Hence, if the Murder rate is high in a state, then Assault
and Rape also tend to be relatively frequent. The same applies to property crimes.
Robbery lies between these neighborhoods, possibly because Robbery may not only
damage the victims' possessions but also their bodies.

This interpretation builds primarily on the first *principal axis*.[1] This axis corresponds to the horizontal dashed line running through the origin of the graph in
Fig. 1.8.

The second principal axis is difficult to interpret. On this axis, Larceny and Robbery are farthest apart. Hence, these two crimes might lead to a meaningful interpretation of the second dimension, but no compelling interpretation seems to offer
itself. This dimension may simply represent the noise of the data. So, one can ask
whether it suffices to represent the given data in a one-dimensional (1d) MDS space.

---

[1]The first principal axis is a straight line which runs through the point cloud so that it is closest
to the points. That is, the sum of the (squared) distances of the points from this line is minimal.
The second principal axis is perpendicular to the first and explains the maximum of the remaining
variance.

The answer to this question is easily found: One simply sets "Dimension = 1" in the GUI in Fig. 1.5, for example, and then repeats the MDS analysis, leaving all other specifications as before.

Figure 1.9 shows the one-dimensional (1d) solution. It closely reproduces the first principal axis of Fig. 1.4. However, its distances correlate with only $r = 0.866$ with the data. Thus, this MDS solution does not represent the data that well. This is also evident from the regression graph in Fig. 1.10. It exhibits clearly more scatter about a linear regression trend than the graph for the two-dimensional (2d) MDS solution in Fig. 1.7. One should, therefore, not interpret this configuration too closely, because it is partly misleading. For example, we note in the data matrix that Robbery and Burglary are correlated with 0.62. We find the same correlation for Robbery and Auto Theft. Yet, in the 1d MDS solution in Fig. 1.9, Burglary is about half as far from Robbery as Auto Theft is from Robbery. So, here we have an example of a noteworthy representation error. On the other hand, this is the largest error, and many of the other data relations are represented quite well. Moreover, the 1d scale makes sense too: It orders the various crimes in terms of increasing violence and brutality.

Table 1.2: Preference rating scores of five persons for four objects, using a 10-point scale (a); embedded into a 9×9 proximity matrix (b); NA = missing data

(a) Preference ratings				
	A	B	C	D
1	3	7	4	9
2	10	8	7	1
3	7	2	5	6
4	8	5	6	7
5	4	7	1	10

(b) Ratings embedded into proximity matrix									
	A	B	C	D	1	2	3	4	5
A	NA	NA	NA	NA	3	10	7	8	4
B	NA	NA	NA	NA	7	8	2	5	7
C	NA	NA	NA	NA	4	7	5	6	1
D	NA	NA	NA	NA	9	1	6	7	10
1	3	7	4	9	NA	NA	NA	NA	NA
2	10	8	7	1	NA	NA	NA	NA	NA
3	7	2	5	6	NA	NA	NA	NA	NA
4	8	5	6	7	NA	NA	NA	NA	NA
5	4	7	1	10	NA	NA	NA	NA	NA

1.2   Basic Ideas of Unfolding

An interesting model that is closely related to MDS is unfolding. While MDS is mostly used to study the proximity structure (often the inter-correlations) of just about any variables, unfolding typically deals with preference data of N persons for n objects and it maps these data *directly* into MDS distances. An unfolding solution, therefore, represents *both* persons and variables in a *joint* space, not just the variables.

We illustrate this with the small example in Table 1.2 (left). It shows preference ratings of persons $1, \ldots, 5$ for objects $A, \ldots, D$ (cars, soft drinks, political parties, or whatever). The scores are on a 10-point scale, where 10 means "my choice", "feel very positive about it", "excellent", etc. We can take Table 1.2 (a) and insert it into a complete proximity matrix as shown in Table 1.2 (b). The cells outside of the data blocks have "NA" entries, because we have no data for the proximities among persons and among objects, respectively.

The matrix in Table 1.2 (b) can be scaled with standard MDS: (1) The MDS representation should have four points for the objects $A, \ldots, D$, and five points for the persons $1, \ldots, 5$; (2) since the data are similarities, we want the model to represent greater data values by smaller distances: A person point should be the closer to an object point, the higher this person rates the object; (3) the NA data impose no restrictions on the MDS solution. For example, the distance between point A and point B can have any value, because it does not represent an observed value. Only the distances among person points and objects points must correspond to given values. Distances within persons and within objects can be chosen arbitrarily.

To find an unfolding solution, we can use the `mds()` function in SMACOF as follows[2]:

```
1  data <- matrix(c(NA,NA,NA,NA,  3,10,  7,  8,  4,
2                    NA,NA,NA,NA,  7,  8,  2,  5,  7,
3                    NA,NA,NA,NA,  4,  7,  5,  6,  1,
4                    NA,NA,NA,NA,  9,  1,  6,  7,10,
5                     3,  7,  4,  9, NA,NA,NA,NA,NA,
6                    10,  8,  7,  1, NA,NA,NA,NA,NA,
7                     7,  2,  5,  6, NA,NA,NA,NA,NA,
8                     8,  5,  6,  7, NA,NA,NA,NA,NA,
9                     4,  7,  1,10, NA,NA,NA,NA,NA), nrow=9, ncol=9)
10 colnames(data) <- c( "A", "B", "C", "D", "1", "2", "3", "4", "5" )
11 diss <- sim2diss(data, method = 10)   # convert ratings into dissimilarities
12 result <- mds(diss, type="ordinal")
13 ## ------------------- Configuration Plot (Fig. 1.11) --------------------
14 plot(result, col="cadetblue", pch=16, label.conf=list(cex=1.5, pos=5),
15     ylim=c(-1.2, 1.2), cex.axis=1.2, cex.lab=1.2,
16     xlab="Dimension 1", ylab="Dimension 2", main="")
17 ## ------------------- Shepard Diagram (Fig. 1.12) --------------------
18 dat <- data[lower.tri(diss)]; dist <- as.vector(result$confdist)
19 dhat <- as.vector(result$dhat)
20 plot(dat, dist, pch=21, cex=2, ylim=c(0.8, 2.5), xlim=c(0, 11),
21     xlab="Preference Ratings", ylab="Distances in Unfolding Space" )
22 points(dat, dhat, pch=16, col="blue"); dat2 <- dat[order(dat, -dhat)]
23 dhat2 <- dhat[order(dat, -dhat)]; lines(dat2, dhat2, col="red")
```

---

[2]The code can be greatly simplified by using `plot(result)` and `plot(result, plot.type = "Shepard")` for plots with default properties. The plots can be modified by various arguments (as in the first plot command). The user can also generate his/her own plots using other R-functions or packages as shown here for the Shepard diagram.

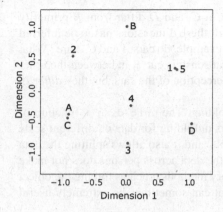
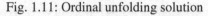

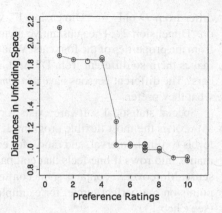

Fig. 1.11: Ordinal unfolding solution

Fig. 1.12: Unfolding distances versus preference data, with monotone regression line

With the commands 1–12, we obtain an almost perfect (ordinal) unfolding solution (Fig. 1.11). That is, the order of the preference data corresponds closely to the order of the distances between person points and object points of the unfolding solution. For example, the observed rating of person 1 for object A is $r(1, A) = 3$, and this is mapped into the unfolding distance $d(1, A) = 1.82$. Moreover, the observed rating $r(5, C) = 1$ corresponds to $d(5, C) = 1.88$. So, $r(1, A) > r(5, C)$ and $d(1, A) < d(5, C)$, which means that these two observations are represented by distances that are properly ordered.

The fit of the unfolding solution to the data is comprehensively shown by the *Shepard diagram*[3] in Fig. 1.12. The plot exhibits that the (data-based) distances of the unfolding solution are nearly (inversely) ordered as the data that they represent. The model fit would be 100% perfect, if all open circles were on a (weakly[4]) monotonically dropping regression line running from left to right.

The points representing the persons in an unfolding solution are often called *ideal points*, because they are the points of maximal preference in space. The closer an object to a person's ideal point, the stronger his/her preference for that object.

What does an unfolding solution tell us? Assume the objects $A, \ldots, D$ in Fig. 1.11 were automobiles. A market researcher may conclude here that the test persons discriminate among these cars using two dimensions: In their perception, A and C

---

[3] A Shepard diagram is a scatter plot of the data versus the MDS/unfolding distances, together with the regression line used in the particular scaling model.

[4] "Weakly" means that the trend line exhibits some horizontal sections. In practice, this is irrelevant, because if you tilt the steps just a little, the regression trend keeps dropping as you move to the right on the X-axis.

differ from D only on "Dimension 1", while A, C, and D differ from B primarily on "Dimension 2". The substantive meaning of these dimensions has to be inferred from the properties of the four cars: What, for example, do cars A and C share? What makes them so different from D? And in what sense is car B in between the other cars? The different persons have a *common* perception of the cars, but they *differ* in what they prefer.

Special statistical software exists for unfolding. The unfolding() function of SMACOF is the most flexible program. It offers unfolding for data on different scale levels (ordinal, interval, and ratio), for example, and it also allows splitting the data matrix into rows if one feels that comparing the data across persons does not make sense. Moreover, it contains some confirmatory methods (such as forcing the object points onto a perfect circle, for example) that can sometimes be extremely useful (see Chap. 8).

Using a special unfolding program not only makes the analysis less cumbersome, but such programs are designed to avoid *degenerate* solutions that can easily result in unfolding because of the big "NA" blocks in the data. For such data, an ordinary MDS program (see, e.g., Fig. 1.5 and the option "Rectangular (unfolding model)") may deliver a solution where all person points lie in one dense cluster, and all object points in another such cluster, or where all person points lie in one point and all objects points are on a circle around this person point, for example. In such solutions, the distances between person points and object points are all practically equal. Thus, they do not differ much from values that are ordered exactly as the data are ordered— whatever the data! Expressed in terms of a Shepard diagram, the regression line is essentially a straight horizontal line. This "representation" of the data is, therefore, *trivial* and *uninformative*.

1.3 Summary

MDS represents proximity data as distances among points in a multidimensional space. The scaling begins with some initial configuration. Its points are then moved iteratively so that the fit of distances and data is improved until no further improvement seems possible. If the fit is good, the MDS solution can be interpreted in terms of content. Unfolding is a special MDS model that represents both the row variables (usually: persons) and the column variables (usually: objects) of a proximity matrix (usually: preference data). For unfolding, special statistical software exists that is easier to use than ordinary MDS programs and that is designed to avoid degenerate solutions.

References

De Leeuw, J., & Mair, P. (2009). Multidimensional scaling using majorization: SMACOF in R. *Journal of Statistical Software*, *31*(3), 1–30. http://www.jstatsoft.org/v31/i03/.
R Development Core Team. (2017). R: A language and environment for statistical computing [Manual]. Vienna, Austria. https://www.R-project.org/.

Chapter 2
The Purpose of MDS and Unfolding

Abstract The different purposes of MDS are explained: MDS for visualizing proximity data; MDS for uncovering latent dimensions; MDS as a psychological theory
about judgments of similarity; MDS for testing structural hypotheses; unfolding as
a psychological theory about judgments of preference.

Keywords Latent dimension · Distance axiom · Minkowski distance · Euclidean
distance · City-block distance · Dominance metric · Partition · Facet · Radex ·
Cylindrex · External unfolding · Internal unfolding

2.1 MDS for Visualizing Proximity Data

In recent years, MDS has mostly been used as a tool for analyzing proximity data of
all kinds (e.g., correlations, similarity ratings, co-occurrence data). Most of all, MDS
serves to visualize such data, making them accessible to the eye of the researcher.
Let us consider a typical application. Figure 2.1 shows a case from industrial psychology. Its 27 points represent 25 items and two indexes from an employee survey
in an international IT company. Two examples for the items are: "All in all, I am
satisfied with my pay," and "I like my work," both employing a Likert-type response
scale ranging from "fully agree" to "fully disagree." The two indexes are scale values that summarize the employees' responses to a number of items that focus on
their affective commitment to the company and on their general job satisfaction,
respectively. The distance between two points in Fig. 2.1 represents (quite precisely)
the correlation of the respective variables. As all variables are non-negatively inter-
correlated, it is particularly easy to interpret this MDS configuration: The closer two
points, the higher the correlation of the variables they represent. Hence, one notes,
for example, that since "satisfied with pay" and "satisfied with benefits" are close
neighbors in the MDS plane (see lower left-hand corner of the plot), employees rated
these issues similarly: Those who were relatively satisfied with one job aspect were
also relatively satisfied with the other aspect. In contrast, being satisfied with pay is
far from "encouraged to voice new ideas" (see top of the plot), and, hence, these two
items are essentially uncorrelated.

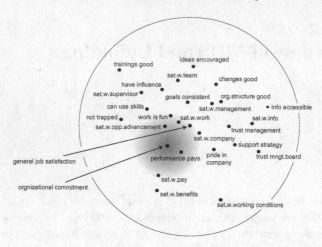

Fig. 2.1 MDS representation of the correlations of 25 items and 2 indexes of an employee survey in an international IT company. The grayed area contains likely drivers of organizational commitment

The value of this MDS configuration is based on the notion that a picture is worth more than a 1,000 words or numbers. Without proper statistical tools, it is impossible to understand the structure among the 27×27 inter-correlation matrix with its 351 coefficients, while the MDS configuration is easy to explore and helpful for guiding data-based discussions.

The fact that 351 correlations can be represented by distances among 27 points that lie in a merely two-dimensional space makes clear, moreover, that the data are highly structured. Random data would require much higher-dimensional spaces. Hence, the persons who answered this employee survey must have generated their answers from a consistent system of attitudes and opinions, and not by generating evasive random ratings.

The ratings also make sense psychologically, because items of similar content are grouped in small neighborhoods of the MDS space. For example, the various items related to management (e.g., trust management, trust management board, support strategy) form such a neighborhood of items that received similar ratings in the survey.

One also notes that the one point that represents general job satisfaction lies somewhere in the central region of the point configuration. This central position reflects the fact that general job satisfaction is positively correlated with each of the 25 items of this survey. Items located more at the border of the MDS plot are substantially and positively correlated with the items in their neighborhood, but not with items opposite of them in the configuration. With them, they are essentially uncorrelated.

The plot leads to many more insights. One notes, for example, that the employees tend to be the more satisfied with their job in general, the more they like their tasks and the more they are satisfied with their opportunities for advancement. Satisfaction with working conditions, in contrast, is a relatively poor predictor of general job satisfaction in this company.

Because the company suffered from high turnover, the variable "commitment to the company" was of particular interest. Management wanted to know what could be done to reduce turnover. The MDS configuration can be explored for answers to this question. One begins by studying the neighborhood of the point representing commitment to the company (see dark cloud around the commitment point in Fig. 2.1), looking for items that offer themselves for action. That is, one attempts to find points close to commitment that received poor ratings and where actions that would improve these ratings appear possible. Expressed in terms of the MDS configuration, this can be understood as grabbing such a point and then pulling it upwards so that the whole plane is lifted like a rubber sheet, first of all in the neighborhood of commitment. Managers understand this notion and, if guided properly, they are able to identify and discuss likely "drivers" of the variable of interest efficiently and effectively. In the given configuration, one notes, for example, that the employees' commitment is strongly correlated with how they feel about their opportunities for advancement (42% satisfied (see Borg 2008, p. 311f.)); with how much they like the work they do (69% like it); with how satisfied they are with the company overall (88% satisfied); and, most of all, with how positive they feel about "performance pays" (only 36% positive). Thus, if one interprets this network of correlations causally, with the variables in the neighborhood of commitment as potential drivers of commitment, it appears that the employees' commitment can be enhanced most effectively by improving the employees' opinions about the performance-dependency of their pay and how they feel about their chances for advancement. Improving other variables, such as the employees' attitudes toward management, is not likely to impact organizational commitment that much.

In this example, MDS serves to visualize the inter-correlations among a set of items. The user is given a natural platform to see, explore, and discuss the structure of these items. This can be particularly useful if the number of items is large, because each additional item adds just one new point to the MDS plot, while it adds as many new coefficients to a correlation matrix as there are variables.

2.2   MDS for Uncovering Latent Dimensions of Judgment

A fundamental question of psychology is how subjective impressions of similarity come about. Why does Julia look like Mike's daughter? How come that a Porsche appears to be more similar to a Ferrari than to a Cadillac? To explain such judgments or perceptions, distance models offer themselves as natural candidates. In such models, the various objects are first conceived as points in a "psychological space" that is *spanned* by the subjective *attributes* of the objects. The distances among the points then serve to generate overall impressions of greater or smaller similarity. Yet, the problem with such models is that one hardly ever knows what attributes a person assigns to the objects under consideration. This is where MDS comes in: With its help, one attempts to infer these attributes from global similarity judgments.

Let us consider an example that is typical for the early days of MDS. Wish (1971) wanted to know the attributes that people use when judging the similarity of different countries. He conducted an experiment where 18 students were asked to rate each pair of 12 different countries on their overall similarity. For these ratings, an answer scale from "extremely dissimilar" (coded as 1) to "extremely similar" (coded as 9) was offered to the respondents. No explanation was given on what was meant by "similar": "There were no instructions concerning the characteristics on which these similarity judgments were to be made; this was information to discover rather than to impose" (Kruskal and Wish 1978, p. 30). The observed similarity ratings, averaged over the 18 respondents, are available in SMACOF, where they can be called by the command data(wish).[1] They are also shown in Table 3.1(lower half) on p. 30.

An MDS analysis of these data with one of the major MDS programs, using the usual default parameters,[2] delivers the solution shown in Fig. 2.2. Older MDS programs generate only the Cartesian coordinates of the points (as shown in Table 2.1 in columns "Dim.1" and "Dim.2," respectively, together called *coordinate matrix* and denoted as **X** in this book). Modern programs also produce graphical output as in Fig. 2.2. The plot shows, for example, that the countries Yugoslavia and USSR are represented by points that are close together. In the data table, we find that the similarity rating on these two countries is relatively high (=6.67, the largest value). So, this relation is properly represented in the MDS plane. In Fig. 2.2, we note further that the points representing Brazil and China are far from each other and that their similarity rating is small (=2.39). Thus, this relation is also properly represented in the MDS solution. Checking more of these correspondences suggests that the MDS solution is a good representation of the similarity data.

If we are willing to accept that the given MDS plane exhibits the essential structure of the similarity data, we can interpret this psychological map. In particular, we now ask what psychologically meaningful "dimensions" span this space. Formally, the map is spanned by what the computer program delivers, i.e., by "Dimension 1" and "Dimension 2." These dimensions are the principal axes of the point configuration. However, one can also *rotate* these dimensions (holding the configuration of points fixed), because any other system of two coordinate axes—even oblique ones—also spans the plane. Hence, one looks for a coordinate system that is psychologically most meaningful. Wish (1971) suggests that rotating the coordinate system in Fig. 2.2 by 45 degrees leads to such dimensions. On the diagonal from the South-West to the North-East corner of Fig. 2.2, Congo, Brazil, and Cuba are on one end, while Japan, Israel, and the USA are on the other end. On the basis of what he knew about these countries, and assuming that the respondents used similar criteria, Wish interpreted

---

[1] Typing data() gives you a listing of all the data sets available in the R packages loaded previously by library(); data(wish) loads the data set wish; help(wish) provides information about wish.

[2] Most MDS programs are set, by default, to deliver a *two-dimensional* solution for data assumed to have an *ordinal* scale level.

Fig. 2.2 MDS representation of mean similarity ratings for twelve countries

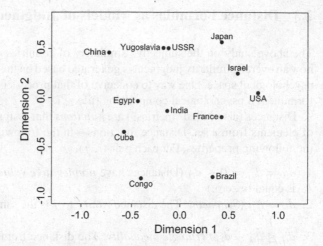

Table 2.1 Coordinates **X** of points in Fig. 2.2; Economic Development and Number of Inhabitants show further measurements on these countries in 1971

Country	No.	X Dim.1	X Dim.2	Economic Development	Number of In-habitants (millions)
Brazil	1	0.33	−0.80	3	87
Congo	2	−0.40	−0.82	1	17
Cuba	3	−0.58	−0.35	3	8
Egypt	4	−0.44	−0.04	3	30
France	5	0.42	−0.20	8	1
India	6	−0.13	−0.13	3	500
Israel	7	0.59	0.25	7	3
Japan	8	0.42	0.57	9	100
China	9	−0.72	0.46	4	750
USSR	10	−0.12	0.51	7	235
USA	11	0.79	0.05	10	201
Yugoslavia	12	−0.17	0.51	6	20

this diagonal as "underdeveloped versus developed." The second dimension, the North-West to the South-East line, was interpreted as "Pro-Communist versus Pro-Western."

These interpretations are meant as hypotheses about the attributes that the respondents (not the researcher!) use when they generate their similarity judgments. That is, the respondents are assumed to look at each pair of countries, compute their differences in terms of Underdeveloped/Developed and Pro-Communist/Pro-Western, respectively, and then derive an overall distance from these two *intra-dimensional* distances. Whether this explanation is indeed valid cannot be checked any further with the given data. MDS only suggests that this is a model that is compatible with the observations.

2.3   Distance Formulas as Models of Judgment

The above study on the subjective similarity of countries does not explain exactly how an overall similarity judgment is generated based on the information given by the psychological space. One way to conceive of that process is to interpret the distance formula as a psychological composition rule.

Distances (also called "metrics") are *functions* that assign a real value to each pair of elements from a set. Distance functions—in the following denoted as d_{ij}—have the following properties. For each pair (i, j),

1. $d_{ii} = d_{jj} = 0 \le d_{ij}$ (Distances have *nonnegative values*; only the self-distance is equal to zero.)
2. $d_{ij} = d_{ji}$ (*Symmetry*: The distance from i to j is the same as the distance from j to i.)
3. $d_{ij} \le d_{ik} + d_{kj}$ (*Triangle inequality*: The distance from i to j via k is at least as large as the direct "path" from i to j.)

One can check if given dissimilarity data for pairs of objects satisfy these properties. If they do, they are distances; if they do not, they are not distances (even though they may be "approximate" distances).

A set M of objects together with a distance function d is called a *metric space*. A special case of a metric space is the Euclidean space. Its distance function does not only satisfy the above distance axioms, but it can also be interpreted geometrically as the distance of the points i and j of a multidimensional Cartesian space. That means that Euclidean distances can be computed from the points' Cartesian coordinates as

$$d_{ij}(\mathbf{X}) = \sqrt{(x_{i1} - x_{j1})^2 + \dots + (x_{im} - x_{jm})^2}, \tag{2.1}$$

$$= \left(\sum_{a=1}^{m} (x_{ia} - x_{ja})^2 \right)^{1/2}, \tag{2.2}$$

where $\mathbf{X}$ denotes a configuration of n points in m-dimensional space, and x_{ia} is the value ("coordinate") of point i on the coordinate axis a. This formula can be generalized to a family of distance functions, the *Minkowski distances*:

$$d_{ij}(\mathbf{X}) = \left(\sum_{a=1}^{m} |x_{ia} - x_{ja}|^p \right)^{1/p}, \quad p \ge 1. \tag{2.3}$$

Setting $p = 2$, formula (2.3) becomes the Euclidean distance. For $p = 1$, one gets the *city-block distance*; for $p \to \infty$, the formula yields the *dominance metric*.

As a model for judgments of (dis-)similarity, the city-block distance ($p = 1$) seems to be the most plausible composition rule, at least in case of "analyzable" stimuli with "obvious and compelling" (Torgerson 1958, p. 254) dimensions. It claims that a person forms a judgment by first assessing the distance of the respective two objects on each of the m dimensions of the psychological space, and then adding these intra-dimensional distances to arrive at an overall rating of dissimilarity.

If one interprets formula (2.3) literally, then it suggests for $p = 2$ that the person first squares each intra-dimensional distance, then sums the resulting values, and finally takes the square root. This appears hardly plausible. However, one can also interpret the formula differently. That is, the parameter p of the distance formula can be seen as a *weight* function: For values of $p > 1$, large intra-dimensional distances have an over-proportional influence on the global judgment, and when $p \to \infty$, only the largest intra-dimensional distance matters. Indeed, for p-values as small as 10, the global distance is almost equal to the largest intra-dimensional distance.[3] Thus, one hypothesis is that when judgments become more difficult (e.g., because of time pressure), persons tend to focus on the largest intra-dimensional distances only. This corresponds, formally, to choosing a large p value.

Another line of argumentation is that city-block composition rules make sense only for analyzable stimuli with their obvious and compelling dimensions (such as geometric figures like rectangles), whereas for "integral" stimuli (such as color patches), the Euclidean distance that expresses the length of the direct path through the psychological space is more adequate (Garner 1974).

Choosing parameters other than $p = 2$ has surprising consequences. It generates geometries that differ substantially from those we are familiar with. What we know, and what is called the *natural* geometry, is Euclidean geometry. It is natural because distances and structures in Euclidean geometry are as they "should" be. A circle, for example, is "round." If $p \neq 1$, circles do not seem to be round. In the city-block plane, a circle *looks* like a square that sits on one of its corners (see left panel of Fig. 2.3). Yet, this geometrical figure *is* indeed a circle, because it is the set of all points that have the same distance from their midpoint M. The reason for its peculiar-looking shape is that the distances of any two points in the city-block plane correspond to the length of a path between these points that can run only in North-South or West-East directions, but never along diagonals—just like walking from A to B in Manhattan, where the distance may be "two blocks West and three blocks North." Hence the name city-block distance. For points that lie on a line parallel to one of the coordinate axes, all Minkowski distances are equal (see points M and i in Fig. 2.3); otherwise, they are not equal. If you walk from M to j (or to j' or j'', respectively) on a Euclidean path ("as the crow flies"), the distance is shorter than choosing the city-block path which runs around the corner. The shortest path corresponds to the dominance distance: The largest intra-dimensional difference will get you from M to the other points. This is important for the MDS user because it shows that rotating the coordinate axes generally changes all Minkowski distances, except Euclidean distances.

---

[3]This is easy to see from an example: If point i has the coordinates $(0, 0)$ and j the coordinates $(3, 2)$, we get the intra-dimensional distances $|0 - 3| = 3$ and $|0 - 2| = 2$, respectively. The overall distance d_{ij}, with $p = 1$, is thus equal to $2 + 3 = 5.00$. For $p = 2$, the overall distance is 3.61. For $p = 10$, it is equal to 3.01.

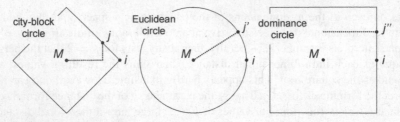

Fig. 2.3 Three circles with the same radius in the city-block plane, the Euclidean plane, and the dominance plane, respectively

To see how the distance formula can serve as a model of judgment, consider an experiment by Borg and Leutner (1983). They constructed rectangles on the basis of the grid design in Fig. 2.4. Each point in this grid defines a rectangle. Rectangle 6, for example, had a width of 4.25 cm and a height of 1.25 cm; rectangle 4 was 3.00 cm wide and 2.75 cm tall. A total of 21 persons rated (twice) the similarity of each pair of these 16 rectangles (see example in Fig. 2.4, lower panel) on a 10-point scale ranging from "0 = equal, identical" to "9 = very different." The means of these ratings over persons and replications is given by calling `data(rectangles)` in the SMACOF package.

The MDS representation (using city-block distances)[4] of these ratings is the grid of solid points in Fig. 2.5. From what we discussed above, we know that this configuration must not be rotated relative to the given coordinate axes, because rotations would *change* its (city-block) distances and, since the MDS representation in Fig. 2.5 is the best-possible data representation, this would deteriorate the correspondence of MDS distances and data.

If one allows for some rescaling of the width and height coordinates of the rectangles, one can fit the design configuration quite well to the MDS configuration (see grid of dashed lines in Fig. 2.5). The rescaling also makes psychological sense: It exhibits a logarithmic shrinkage of the grid lines from left to right and from bottom to top, as expected by psychophysical theory.

The deviations of the rescaled design grid from the MDS configuration do not seem to be systematic. Hence, one may conclude that the subjects did indeed generate their ratings by a composition rule described by the city-block distance formula (including a logarithmic rescaling of intra-dimensional distances according to the Weber–Fechner law). The MDS solution also shows that differences in the rectangles' heights are psychologically more important for similarity judgments than differences in the rectangles' widths.

---

[4]The solution was computed with SYSTAT. Neither PROXSCAL nor SMACOF offer city-block distances. In SYSTAT, the city-block metric is invoked by setting the "R-metric:" option in the GUI in Fig. 1.5 equal to "1".

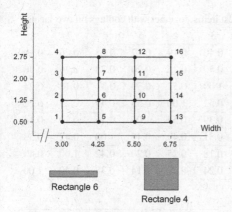

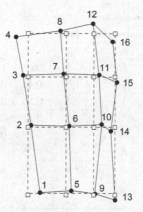

Fig. 2.4 Design configuration for 16 rectangles with different widths and heights; lower panel shows two rectangles in a pair comparison

Fig. 2.5 MDS configuration with cityblock distances for rectangle similarity data (points) and design configuration of Fig. 2.4 (squares) fitted to MDS configuration

2.4 MDS for Testing Structural Hypotheses

A frequent application of MDS is testing structural hypotheses. A typical case is intelligence diagnostics (Guttman and Levy 1991). Here, persons are asked to solve several test items. The items can be classified on the basis of their content into different categories of two design factors, called *facets* in this context. Some test items require the testee to solve computational problems with *numbers* and numerical operations. Other items ask for *geometrical* solutions where figures have to be rotated in three-dimensional space or pictures have to be completed. Other test items require *applying* learned rules, while still others have to be solved by *finding* such rules. One can always code test items in terms of such facets, but the facets are truly interesting only if they exert some control over the observations, i.e., if the distinctions they make are mirrored somehow in corresponding effects on the data side. The data in our small example are the inter-correlations of eight intelligence test items shown in Table 2.2. The items are coded in terms of the facets "Format = {N(umerical), G(eometrical)}" and "Requirement = {A(pply), I(nfer)}".

A 2d MDS representation of the data in Table 2.2 is shown in Fig. 2.6. We now ask whether the facets Format and Requirement surface in some way in this plane. For the facet Format, we find that the plane can indeed be *partitioned* by a straight line such that all points labeled as "G" are on one side, and all "N" points on the other (Fig. 2.7). Similarly, using the codings for the facet Requirement, the plane can be partitioned into two subregions, an A- and an I-region. For the Requirement facet, we have drawn the partitioning line in a curved way, anticipating test items of a third kind on this facet: Guttman and Levy (1991) extend the facet Requirement by adding the element "Learning." They also extend the facet Format by adding "Verbal."

Table 2.2 Inter-correlations of eight intelligence test items, together with codings on two facets

Format	Requirement	Item	1	2	3	4	5	6	7	8
N	A	1	1.00	0.67	0.40	0.19	0.12	0.25	0.26	0.39
N	A	2	0.67	1.00	0.50	0.26	0.20	0.28	0.26	0.38
N	I	3	0.40	0.50	1.00	0.52	0.39	0.31	0.18	0.24
G	I	4	0.19	0.26	0.52	1.00	0.55	0.49	0.25	0.22
G	I	5	0.12	0.20	0.39	0.55	1.00	0.46	0.29	0.14
G	A	6	0.25	0.28	0.31	0.49	0.46	1.00	0.42	0.38
G	A	7	0.26	0.26	0.18	0.25	0.29	0.42	1.00	0.40
G	A	8	0.39	0.38	0.24	0.22	0.14	0.38	0.40	1.00

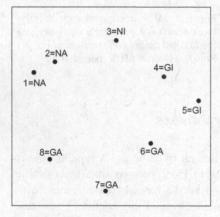

Fig. 2.6 MDS solution for correlations in Table 2.2

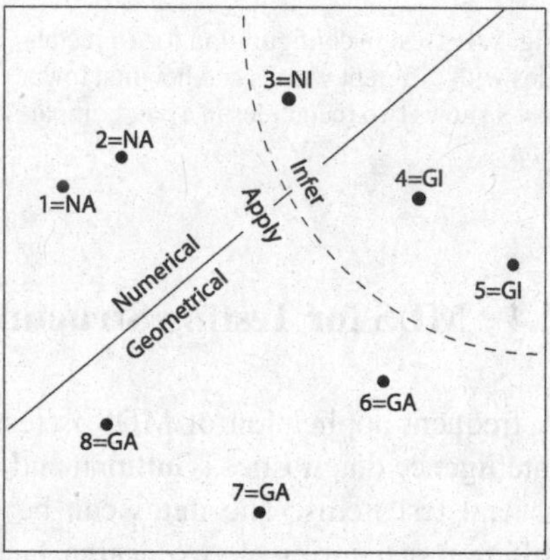

Fig. 2.7 MDS configuration partitioned by two facets

For the inter-correlations of items in this extended 3×3 design, that is, for items coded in terms of two 3-element facets, MDS leads to structures with a partitioning system as shown in Fig. 2.8. This pattern, termed *radex*, is often found for items that combine a qualitative facet (such as Format) and an ordered facet (such as Requirement). For the universe of typical intelligence test items, Guttman and Levy (1991) suggest yet another facet, called Communication. It distinguishes among Oral, Manual, and Paper-and-Pencil items. If there are test items of all $3 \times 3 \times 3$ types, MDS leads to a three-dimensional *cylindrex* structure as shown in Fig. 2.9. Such a cylindrex shows, for example, that items of the Infer type have relatively high inter-correlations (given a certain mode of Communication), irrespective of their Format. It is interesting to see that Apply is "in between" Infer and Learn. We also note that our small sample of test items of Table 2.2 fits perfectly into the larger structure of the universe of intelligence test items.

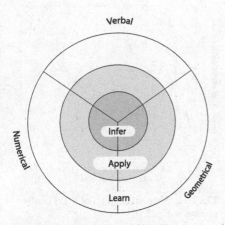

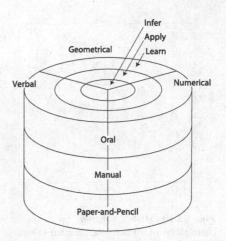

Fig. 2.8 Schematic radex of intelligence test items

Fig. 2.9 Cylindrex of intelligence test items

A more recent example of using MDS to test structural hypotheses is a study by Borg et al. (2017).[5] They asked 151 US adults to answer the PVQ40, a questionnaire that measures the personal importance of ten basic values (PO = power, AC = achievement, HE = hedonism, ST = stimulation, SD = self-direction, UN = universalism, BE = benevolence, TR = tradition, CO = conformity, and SE = security). The PVQ consists of 40 items, each a short portrait of one person. Each portrait describes a person's goals, aspirations, and desires that reflect that person's values. Participants rate the extent to which each person portrayed is similar to themselves, using a 6-point response scale ranging from "not like me at all" (0) to "very much like me" (6).

Value researchers typically first inter-correlate the scores of such items and then run ordinal MDS on the correlations. This leads to Fig. 2.10, computed by SMACOF (see the R script on p. 22). It represents the correlations among the items rather precisely, as can be seen by the relatively small scatter about the regression line in Fig. 2.11. The 40 points in Fig. 2.10 are labeled here in terms of the basic values that the items are measuring. For example, co1 is item 1 of the PVQ measuring conformity, and po2 is item 2 assessing power. To facilitate interpretation, a set of straight lines was added here by hand. These lines cut ("partition") the space like a cake into wedge-like regions. The partitioning lines form a particular pattern called *circumplex*, a circle of regions emanating from a common origin. Each region contains only items of one particular type—except for a few minor errors where points (e.g., co4 or tr1) fall into the respective neighboring region. Such a structure

---

[5]The data set is contained in SMACOF. It is loaded automatically when calling SMACOF. You can check it by typing `attributes(PVQ40)` or `head(PVQ40)`, for example. There is no need to explicitly load the data by typing `data(PVQ40)`, but it would give you an error message if a file with this name does not exist.

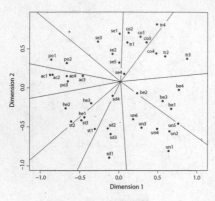

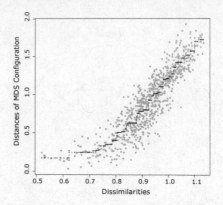

Fig. 2.10 MDS solution of inter-correlations of 40 items on personal values with circumplex partitioning

Fig. 2.11 Shepard diagram of MDS configuration in Fig. 2.10

is certainly *unlikely* to result by chance, and this is even more true since it *replicates* numerous similar studies.

Another way to look at the MDS solution is checking to what extent items constructed to measure the same construct appear homogeneous. This analysis can be made easier by drawing convex hulls around items that belong to the same category (Fig. 2.12). Since all items are coded here as se1, co2, etc., we can generate such a plot as follows[6]:

```
1  r <- cor(PVQ40, use="pairwise.complete.obs")
2  diss <- sim2diss(r, method="corr")
3  res <- mds(delta=diss, type="ordinal")  ## ordinal MDS
4  codes <- substring(colnames(PVQ40), 1, 2)
5  plot(res, main="", hull.conf=list(hull=TRUE, ind=codes, col="coral1", lwd=2))
```

Rather   than scaling items, one could first average the various item ratings to yield importance indexes for each of the ten basic values, and then run an MDS on the 10×10 inter-correlation matrix of these index scores[7]:

---

[6]Note that we use the first two characters of the variables' codes (i.e., "se", "co", etc.) in ind=codes to group the points.

[7]We show here how this is done, but the result is also directly available in SMACOF in the file PVQ40agg.

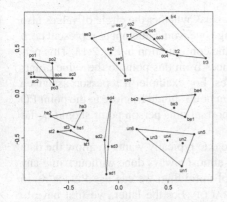

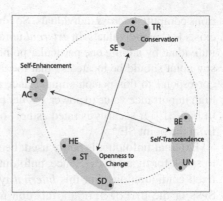

Fig. 2.12 MDS solution of personal values with convex hulls surrounding items measuring the same construct

Fig. 2.13 MDS configuration of ten indexes on basic personal values; double-arrowed lines show two oppositions; circle optimally fitted to points

```
1  SE <- rowMeans(subset(PVQ40, select=c(se1,se2)), na.rm=TRUE)
2  CO <- rowMeans(subset(PVQ40, select=c(co1,co2)), na.rm=TRUE)
3  TR <- rowMeans(subset(PVQ40, select=c(tr1,tr2)), na.rm=TRUE)
4  BE <- rowMeans(subset(PVQ40, select=c(be1,be2)), na.rm=TRUE)
5  UN <- rowMeans(subset(PVQ40, select=c(un1,un2,un3)), na.rm=TRUE)
6  SD <- rowMeans(subset(PVQ40, select=c(sd1,sd2)), na.rm=TRUE)
7  ST <- rowMeans(subset(PVQ40, select=c(st1,st2)), na.rm=TRUE)
8  HE <- rowMeans(subset(PVQ40, select=c(he1,he2)), na.rm=TRUE)
9  AC <- rowMeans(subset(PVQ40, select=c(ac1,ac2)), na.rm=TRUE)
10 PO <- rowMeans(subset(PVQ40, select=c(po1,po2)), na.rm=TRUE)
11 raw <- cbind(SE,CO,TR,BE,UN,SD,ST,HE,AC,PO)
12 R <- cor(raw); diss <- sim2diss(R, method="corr")
13 result <- mds(diss, type="ordinal"); plot(result)
14 out <- fitCircle(result$conf[,1], result$conf[,2])
15 draw.circle(out$cx, out$cy, radius=out$radius, border="black", lty=2)
```

Figure 2.13 shows that this analysis yields a simple pattern: The ten value points are close to a circle fitted to the point configuration using the `fitCircle()` function. Moreover, the order of the points on this circle replicates what many other studies have found. Figure 2.13 also exhibits an interpretation in terms of two bipolar directions: self-enhancement versus self-transcendence, and openness to change versus conservation.

2.5 Unfolding as a Psychological Model of Preference

Let us continue with the above data set on personal values, but now analyze it by unfolding. Unfolding stays closer to the data, and individuals are not lost in correlations computed *across* individuals. So, one can ask whether the circle of values also exists *within* individuals. In *external* unfolding, we would attempt to represent each individual by adding one particular point to the configuration in Fig. 2.13. This person point should be located so that the distances from this point to the value points correspond to this person's importance scores. For example, if a person assigns a high importance value to power, his/her person point should be close to the point PO in Fig. 2.13. If security is rated as not so important, this person point should be far from the point SE.[8]

External unfolding is rarely used, because one typically wants to allow the data to speak for themselves. Hence, unfolding is almost always done without using any fixed configurations. For this *internal* type of unfolding, we can use PREFSCAL in SPSS or the `unfolding()` function in SMACOF. For the latter, we first have to reverse the importance scores by turning them into dissimilarities.[9] Dissimilarities can be produced by subtracting each importance score from the largest observed importance score. We then search for a configuration with 10 points for the 10 basic values and with 146 additional points for the 146 individuals such that the distances between the person points and the value points directly match the dissimilarities (except for an overall scaling factor).[10] The commands for this job are[11]:

```
1  c <- PVQ40agg - rowMeans(PVQ40agg) ## center ratings
2  diss <- max(c) - c ## turn preference ratings into dissimilarities
3  result <- unfolding(diss)
4  plot(result,
5    pch = 16, cex=2, main="",
6    col.columns="black", label.conf.columns = list(pos=3, col=1, cex=1.5),
7    col.rows = "red", label.conf.rows = list(pos=1, col="red", cex=1) )
8  para <- fitCircle(result$conf.col[,1], result$conf.col[,2])
9  draw.circle(para$cx, para$cy, radius=para$radius, border="blue", lty=2)
```

Figures 2.14 and 2.15 show the results. The points representing the ten personal values PO, ... , SE lie close to a circle (dashed line). They also form certain basic oppositions ("higher-order values"), i.e., self-enhancement (PO, AC) versus self-transcendence (BE, UN) and openness to change (HE, ST, SD) versus conservation (TR, CO, SE), as predicted by Schwartz (1992). Indeed, even their order on the circle supports the theory.

The persons are represented in Fig. 2.14 by the points labeled with the row numbers of the data matrix. Almost every person is well represented in this configuration. That is not trivial, because, for example, a person who rates achievement as not so

---

[8]Expressed more formally, in external unfolding either the person points or the object points are *fixed* and the other points are then optimally fitted into this fixed point configuration.

[9]We here also first center each person's ratings, i.e., subtract the mean of his/her ratings from his/her rating scores to generate "relative value priorities." This leads to a simpler model by reducing the dimensionality of the solution. See Sect. 8.1.

[10]This model is *ratio* unfolding. This is the default of the `unfolding()` function.

[11]You can generate a nice plot by simply typing `plot(result)`. We here show some ways to customize such plots. You can also use R graphics or special graphics packages for customized plotting. However, SMACOF offers some easy-to-use arguments for plotting convex hulls (see Fig. 2.12) or confidence regions of the points (see Fig. 3.8) that are particularly useful in the MDS context.

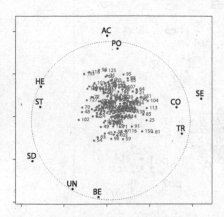

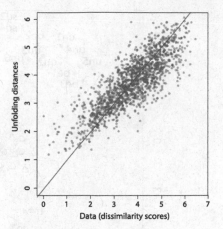

Fig. 2.14 Unfolding solution of PVQ40 data; numbers represent persons; circle optimally fitted to points representing personal values

Fig. 2.15 Shepard diagram of unfolding distances versus reversed importance ratings (dissimilarities)

important but power as very important would *not* fit well into this solution, because this person's profile would require a point that is far from AC but close to PO. Such a point obviously does not exist in Fig. 2.14, because AC and PO are close together and, thus, must receive similar ratings.

We can also run an unfolding job on all 40 items rather than on only 10 indexes derived from these items. This allows a more detailed study. In particular, we can check the homogeneity of the indexes. To run this job, we use the commands in the box on p. 26 below.

We thus obtain Fig. 2.16 where the persons points are displayed by triangles (men) or by circles (women). We first note that when rotating this configuration by about 60 degrees counter-clockwise, it becomes easier to compare it to Fig. 2.14, because then the points that relate to AC, for example, move to the top of the plot, and those measuring UN and BE to the left lower corner of the box. The overall orientation of an MDS plot is not determined by the data and, therefore, substantively meaningless.

When taking a closer look at Fig. 2.16, we see that the items in some categories (e.g., TR) scatter quite a bit in space, while others (e.g., PO) form dense clusters. Also, there is considerable overlap of the various types of value items (e.g., BE and UN). This indicates that the circle of 10 basic values may be understood more as a *continuum* of personal values with gradual transitions rather than as a necklace of discrete points.

One can also take a closer look at the distribution of the person points in the unfolding solution. For example, one can ask whether men and women can be discriminated in this space, and how age shows up in the configuration of person points. These questions can be answered by using the dimensions of the unfolding space as

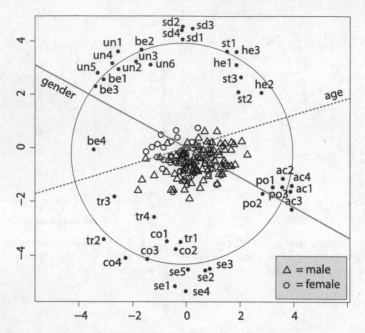

Fig. 2.16 Unfolding solution for 40 items measuring personal values; open circles/triangles represent female/male persons; dashed line optimally represents persons' age; solid line is the discriminant for gender

predictors of the dependent variables gender and age, respectively, as in the following script:

```
1  data.r <- na.omit(PVQ40) ## eliminate persons with missing values
2  data1 <- data.r - rowMeans(data.r)  ## center ratings
3  diss <- max(data1)-data1; unf <- unfolding(diss)
4  plot(unf, what="columns", col.columns=1,
5      label.conf.columns=list(col="black"), main="")
6  ## external variables --------------------------------------------------------
7  gender <- attr(data.r, "Gender")[-attr(data.r, "na.action")]
8  points(unf$conf.row, pch=gender, cex=1.5, lwd=2) ## pch by gender
9  circle <- fitCircle(unf$conf.col[,1], unf$conf.col[,2])
10 draw.circle(circle[[1]], circle[[2]], radius=circle[[3]])
11 ## discriminant analysis for gender ------------------------------------------
12 require(MASS); Y <- unf$conf.row; z <- as.data.frame(cbind(gender, Y))
13 fit <- lda(gender ~ Y, na.action="na.omit", data=z) ## discriminant gender
14 abline(a=0, b=fit$scaling[2]/fit$scaling[1], lty=1, col="red")
15 LDS <- as.data.frame(predict(fit)); L4 <- LDS[,4]
16 tt <- t.test(L4 ~ gender); tt ## t-test for gender discrimination
17 ## multiple regression for age -----------------------------------------------
18 age <- attr(rr, "Age")[-attr(data.r, "na.action")]
19 f <- lm(age ~ Y[,1]+Y[,2])
20 wy <- f$coefficients[3]; wx <- f$coefficients[2]
21 slope <- wy/wx; abline(a=0, b=slope, lty=2, col="blue")
22 age.pred <- predict(f); r <- cor(age, age.pred ); r ## fit of age line
```

The dashed line represents the persons' age in the unfolding plot. The projections of the persons onto this line are correlated with their age with $r = .41$. So, older respondents tend to lean more toward TR and CO, and younger ones more toward ST/HE and PO/AC, a typical finding in value research. The other line is the discriminant for gender. This is the line on which females and males are best separated. Females tend to lie significantly more at the BE/UN end of this scale, and men closer to PO/AC—also normal in value research.

2.6 Summary

MDS started as a psychological model of how persons arrive at judgments of similarity. The model claims that the objects of interest can be understood as points in psychological (i, j) space spanned by the objects' subjective attributes, and that similarity judgments are generated by computing the distance between points. Today, MDS is used primarily for visualizing proximity data so that their structure becomes accessible to the researcher's eye for exploration or for testing. Structural hypotheses are often based on content-based classifications of the variables of interest. Such classifications should surface in the MDS space in corresponding (ordered or unordered) regions. Unfolding is even more psychology-based: It represents both persons and objects as points in a joint space such that the distances between each person's point and each object point represent the observed preference data.

References

Borg, I. (2008). *Employee surveys in management: Theories, tools, and practical applications.* Cambridge, MA: Hogrefe.

Borg, I., Bardi, A., & Schwartz, S. (2017). Does the value circle exist within persons or only across persons? *Journal of Personality, 85*, 151–162.

Borg, I., & Leutner, D. (1983). Dimensional models for the perception of rectangles. *Perception and Psychophysics, 34*, 257–269.

Garner, W. R. (Ed.). (1974). *The processing of information and structure.* Potomac, MD: Erlbaum.

Guttman, L., & Levy, S. (1991). Two structural laws for intelligence tests. *Intelligence, 15*, 79–103.

Kruskal, J. B., & Wish, M. (1978). *Multidimensional scaling.* Beverly Hills, CA: Sage.

Schwartz, S. H. (1992). Universals in the content and structure of values: Theoretical advances and empirical tests in 20 countries. *Advances in Experimental Social Psychology, 25*, 1–65.

Torgerson, W. S. (1958). *Theory and methods of scaling.* New York: Wiley.

Wish, M. (1971). Individual differences in perceptions and preferences among nations. In C. W. King & D. Tigert (Eds.), *Attitude research reaches new heights* (pp. 312–328). Chicago: American Marketing Association.

Chapter 3
The Fit of MDS and Unfolding Solutions

Abstract Ways to assess the goodness of an MDS solution are discussed. The Stress measure is defined as an index that aggregates representation errors. Criteria for evaluating Stress are presented. Stress per Point (SPP) is defined as a way to assess the fit of single points.

Keywords Representation error · Stress · Disparity · Shepard diagram · Stress-1 Stress norm · SPP

3.1 The Global Stress of MDS Solutions

We visualized the goodness of MDS and unfolding solutions above through Shepard diagrams, i.e., scatterplots of the data versus the distances that represent these data in the model. Figure 3.1 gives another example, this one for the MDS representation in Fig. 2.2 of the mean similarity ratings on twelve countries. To understand this diagram in detail, we first look at the data that it represents.

Fig. 3.1 Shepard diagram for the MDS solution in Fig. 2.2

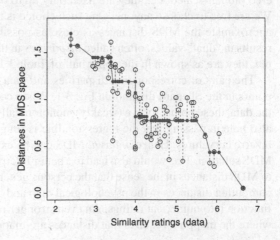

Table 3.1 Data (lower half) and dhats (upper half)

	Bra	Con	Cub	Egy	Fra	Ind	Isr	Jap	Chi	USS	USA	Yug
Brazil	–	0.775	0.775	1.192	0.775	0.775	1.190	1.192	1.705	1.449	0.775	1.449
Congo	4.83	–	0.775	0.775	1.071	0.775	1.449	1.449	1.190	1.400	1.577	1.192
Cuba	5.28	4.56	–	0.775	0.816	0.816	1.192	1.449	0.775	0.775	1.449	0.775
Egypt	3.44	5.00	5.17	–	0.775	0.436	0.775	1.190	0.775	0.775	1.449	0.775
France	4.72	4.00	4.11	4.78	–	1.19	0.816	0.816	1.192	0.775	0.436	0.775
India	4.50	4.83	4.00	5.83	3.44	–	0.816	0.775	0.816	0.775	0.816	0.816
Israel	3.83	3.33	3.61	4.67	4.00	4.11	–	0.775	1.449	0.816	0.436	0.775
Japan	3.50	3.39	2.94	3.83	4.22	4.50	4.83	–	0.816	0.775	0.436	0.775
China	2.39	4.00	5.50	4.39	3.67	4.11	3.00	4.17	–	0.628	1.577	0.775
USSR	3.06	3.39	5.44	4.39	5.06	4.50	4.17	4.61	5.72	–	0.775	0.054
USA	5.39	2.39	3.17	3.33	5.94	4.28	5.94	6.06	2.56	5.00	–	1.192
Yugosl.	3.17	3.50	5.11	4.28	4.72	4.00	4.44	4.28	5.06	6.67	3.56	–

The distances among the points in the MDS solution are exhibited numerically in the upper half of Table 3.2. The data are in the lower half of Table 3.1. Data and distances should be closely related in the sense of the MDS model. Since we chose an ordinal MDS model here, the relationship should be monotonic, and this is roughly the case for the 66 open circles in the Shepard diagram in Fig. 3.1. Each of these circles represents one of the 66 data elements and its corresponding distance in the MDS solution. For example, the mean rating for the pair Brazil–Congo (4.83) is represented by the distance 0.775 between the points Brazil and Congo in Fig. 2.2. Or, the most extreme rating of similarity (6.67, for the pair USSR and Yugoslavia) corresponds to the MDS distance 0.054 (the smallest distance among the points).

To quantify this relationship uniquely, we first note that since the data are considered ordinal-scaled, i,e., they are fixed only up to order-preserving transformations. We are free to choose anyone. One such choice is to rescale the data such that they approximate the MDS distances as close as possible in a least-square sense. This results in "dhat" values, often called *disparities* in the MDS literature. For our example, they are as shown in the upper half of Table 3.1.

The pairs of corresponding disparities and data are displayed by the small solid points in the Shepard diagram in Fig. 3.1. When connected by a line in the order of the data, these points form a (weakly) monotonically descending regression line. We also note in passing that the regression line is roughly linear, with no wild steps or bizarre curvatures. Hence, *interval* MDS can be expected to produce a very similar MDS solution. This would also lead to a better interpretable relation of similarity data to MDS distances in the sense that the persons generate their similarity judgments by computing distances in the psychological map and then map them by a simple linear function into numerical ratings. An even stronger model would be to do *ratio* MDS where the mapping requires that distances are mapped proportionally into ratings.

Table 3.2 Representaion errors (lower half) and distances (upper half)

	Bra	Con	Cub	Egy	Fra	Ind	Isr	Jap	Chi	USS	USA	Yug
Brazil	–	0.737	1.017	1.088	0.612	0.814	1.08	1.372	1.647	1.384	0.966	1.404
Congo	0.001	–	0.500	0.783	1.034	0.734	1.454	1.613	1.316	1.352	1.475	1.344
Cuba	0.058	0.076	–	0.342	1.011	0.492	1.306	1.355	0.821	0.967	1.423	0.945
Egypt	0.011	0.000	0.187	–	0.876	0.321	1.062	1.051	0.572	0.626	1.231	0.603
France	0.026	0.001	0.038	0.010	–	0.559	0.473	0.764	1.323	0.888	0.441	0.923
India	0.002	0.002	0.105	0.013	0.400	–	0.814	0.896	0.840	0.64	0.941	0.643
Israel	0.012	0.000	0.013	0.082	0.118	0.000	–	0.358	1.329	0.752	0.286	0.802
Japan	0.032	0.027	0.009	0.019	0.003	0.015	0.174	–	1.155	0.548	0.635	0.600
China	0.003	0.016	0.002	0.041	0.017	0.001	0.014	0.114	–	0.607	1.571	0.555
USSR	0.004	0.002	0.037	0.022	0.013	0.018	0.004	0.051	0.000	–	1.019	0.052
USA	0.036	0.010	0.001	0.047	0.000	0.016	0.023	0.040	0.000	0.060	–	1.067
Yugosl.	0.002	0.023	0.029	0.029	0.022	0.030	0.001	0.031	0.048	0.000	0.016	–

If the MDS solution were perfect, then all open circles in the Shepard diagram in Fig. 3.1 would lie on the monotonic regression line, because then all data would be mapped into distances that are (weakly) ordered as the data. This is obviously not true here. We can measure "how untrue" it is by considering the squared difference of each disparity and its MDS distance. These *representation errors* are shown in the lower half of Table 3.2. Each of them corresponds to a distance in the Shepard diagram in Fig. 3.1, namely the (squared) vertical distance between an open circle and a solid point on the regression line.

One can see in Table 3.2 that most errors are quite small, with some exceptions. In particular, the pair Egypt and Cuba has a representation error of 0.187, and the one for France versus India is even larger (0.400). Thus, some similarity judgments are relatively poorly represented in MDS space or, expressed differently, in the psychological map of the various countries. This could have many reasons. For example, the students who made the similarity judgments (back in the 1970's) did not know on what criteria they should compare these pairs of countries ("France and Egypt? What do they have in common?"), while in other cases they would use geographical closeness, population size, or political alignment as a basis for comparison. Or the students did not agree on these countries so that when aggregating the data across individuals, we get inconsistencies.

We can construct a global measure of fit (actually: misfit) from these data by simply aggregating the squares of the representation errors (e_{ij}). This is called the *raw Stress* (σ_{raw}). In order to avoid having to write everything twice for dissimilarities and also for similarities, assume that the proximities are given as dissimilarities (δ_{ij}). If the proximities are similarities s_{ij}, they first need to be transformed into dissimilarities (either "by hand" or within the MDS program). A simple scale reversal is accomplished by $\delta_{ij} = c - s_{ij}$, where $c = \max_{ij}(s_{ij})$. A second way of transforming s_{ij} into δ_{ij} exists if all $s_{ij} > 0$. Then choosing $\delta_{ij} = 1/s_{ij}$ is often a good choice. In case of correlations r_{ij}, we can use $\delta_{ij} = (1-r_{ij})^{1/2}$, a conversion turning correlations into Euclidean distances.[1]

Now, assuming that the data are dissimilarities (δ_{ij}),

$$\sigma^2_{raw} = \sum_{i<j} e^2_{ij} = \sum_{i<j} \left(f(\delta_{ij}) - d_{ij}(\mathbf{X}) \right)^2, \qquad (3.1)$$

where $f()$ is the regression function[2] of the MDS model.[3] Missing δ_{ij}'s are skipped in formula 3.1 when summing. The $d_{ij}(\mathbf{X})$'s are distances (computed by formula 2.3 for the configuration $\mathbf{X}$). The $f(\delta_{ij})$'s are disparities, often written as $\widehat{d}_{ij}$'s and, therefore, also called "dhat's". Disparities are computed by regression (of type f) of the dissimilarities onto the distances so that $f(p_{ij}) = \widehat{d}_{ij}$ while minimizing (3.1). The distances $d_{ij}(\mathbf{X})$ are Euclidean distances in almost all MDS applications, computed by formula (2.1).

Since (3.1) is minimized over both $\mathbf{X}$ and the $\widehat{d}_{ij}$'s, an obvious but trivial solution is to choose $\mathbf{X} = \mathbf{0}$ and all $\widehat{d}_{ij} = 0$. To avoid this, (3.1) needs to be normalized. This can be done by dividing (3.1) by the sum of the squared distances. Doing so and taking the square root[4] gives the usual Stress-1 loss function of MDS:

$$\text{Stress-1} = \sqrt{\sum_{i<j} \left(\widehat{d}_{ij} - d_{ij}(\mathbf{X}) \right)^2 / \sum_{i<j} d^2_{ij}(\mathbf{X})}. \qquad (3.2)$$

This normalization has the important consequence that the Stress values do not depend on the size of configuration $\mathbf{X}$ and, therefore, can be compared across different MDS solutions.

So, turning to Table 3.1, the sum of the elements in the lower half of the table is the numerator of Stress-1: $0.001 + 0.058 + \cdots + 0.000 = 2.26$. The sum of the squared elements of the upper half is the denominator: $0.737^2 + 1.017^2 + \cdots + 1.067^2 = 63.74$. Hence, Stress-1 $= (2.26/63.74)^{1/2} = 0.188$.

In Eq. 3.1 for the raw Stress, we added that missing δ_{ij}'s would be skipped. We can express this more formally and more generally as

---

[1] Transformations that convert similarity data into dissimilarities can be done in SMACOF by the function.sim2diss(). For example, if the data is given as the correlation matrix $\mathbf{R}$, diss <- sim2diss(R, method = "corr") will generate a dissimilarity matrix that can be used in out <- mds(diss) to compute an MDS representation.

[2] So, for example, in ratio MDS $f(\delta_{ij}) = b \cdot \delta_{ij}$, where b ($\neq 0$) is a global scaling factor. In interval MDS, $f(\delta_{ij}) = a + b \cdot \delta_{ij}$, where the additive constant a and the multiplicative constant b are picked so that the Stress is minimized. In ordinal MDS, $f()$ is required to be monotonic.

[3] Note that the sum $\sum_{i<j}$ runs over the lower triangular part of the dissimilarities only, because it is assumed that the data are *symmetric* as, for example, in case of Tables 1.1 and 3.1. Asymmetric data require special models. See Sect. 5.4.

[4] The square root has no deeper meaning here; its purpose is to make the resulting values less condensed by introducing more scatter.

$$\sigma_{\text{raw}}^2(\mathbf{X}) = \sum_{i<j} w_{ij} \left(f(\delta_{ij}) - d_{ij}(\mathbf{X}) \right)^2, \tag{3.3}$$

where w_{ij} are nonnegative fixed weights. Such weights can be used to handle missing data by setting $w_{ij} = 0$ for any missing δ_{ij}. However, the weights can also be used to reduce or to increase the influence of each datum on the MDS solution. For example, they can express different reliabilities of the data, or different degrees of certainty in case of direct similarity ratings for pairs of points. They could also be a function of the δ_{ij}'s themselves. For example, one may want to weight the influence of the data by their size so that large dissimilarities have more impact on the MDS solution than small ones. One way to do that is setting $w_{ij} = \delta_{ij}$.

The weights have to be inserted into the denominator of the Stress formula too, and so the formula for Stress-1 becomes

$$\text{Stress-1} = \left(\frac{\sum_{i<j} w_{ij} \left(\widehat{d}_{ij} - d_{ij}(\mathbf{X}) \right)^2}{\sum_{i<j} w_{ij} d_{ij}^2(\mathbf{X})} \right)^{1/2}. \tag{3.4}$$

When using MDS, Stress-1 is almost always reported (and requested by journal editors) as a fit index. Hence, when reading "Stress" in MDS publications, it can be assumed to mean "Stress-1". Other varieties of Stress exist too, but they are not used anymore in practice (Borg and Groenen 2005).

3.2 Evaluating Stress Statistically

A perfect MDS solution has Stress $= 0$. If this is true then the distances of the MDS configuration represent the data without any errors. The MDS solution in Fig. 2.2 has a Stress value of 0.19. Hence, it represents the data only *approximately* in the desired sense. But is this *good enough*? What is often considered as the "nullest of all null" criteria to answer this question is that the observed Stress must be clearly smaller than the Stress value expected for random data. If this is not true, then it is impossible to interpret the MDS distances in any meaningful sense because then the distances are not reliably related to the data. In other words: The points in MDS space are not fixed; rather, they can be moved around more or less arbitrarily without affecting the Stress.

One way to benchmark Stress values is to ask what Stress values can be expected when scaling random data. This is easily answered by running MDS analyses for many (500, say) $n \times n$ proximity matrices with elements sampled from a uniform random distribution and then computing the mean and other statistics of the resulting Stress values for m dimensions (Spence and Ogilvie 1973). SMACOF provides a function that allows the user to compute the expected Stress for any particular combination of parameters: randomstress(n, ndim, nrep, type = c("ratio", "interval", "ordinal", "mspline")). So, for a solu-

Table 3.3 Random Stress norms (mean, 5th percentile) for ordinal, interval, and ratio MDS in 2 or 3 dimensions with 10, . . . , 100 points

Points	Ordinal MDS				Interval MDS				Ratio MDS			
	2-dim.		3-dim.		2-dim.		3-dim.		2-dim.		3-dim.	
n	mean	5%	mean	5%	mean	5%	mean	5%	mean	5%	av	5%
10	0.191	0.154	0.103	0.073	0.236	0.202	0.141	0.116	0.328	0.258	0.298	0.228
15	0.262	0.239	0.169	0.151	0.289	0.268	0.193	0.175	0.383	0.341	0.347	0.301
20	0.298	0.283	0.205	0.192	0.319	0.305	0.222	0.211	0.417	0.385	0.376	0.342
25	0.322	0.311	0.228	0.219	0.337	0.327	0.241	0.233	0.440	0.416	0.397	0.371
30	0.338	0.329	0.244	0.237	0.349	0.342	0.254	0.248	0.457	0.437	0.411	0.392
35	0.349	0.342	0.256	0.250	0.359	0.353	0.264	0.259	0.469	0.452	0.425	0.407
40	0.358	0.353	0.265	0.260	0.366	0.361	0.272	0.268	0.480	0.465	0.435	0.418
45	0.365	0.360	0.273	0.268	0.372	0.367	0.278	0.275	0.489	0.476	0.443	0.430
50	0.371	0.367	0.278	0.274	0.376	0.373	0.283	0.280	0.496	0.484	0.451	0.440
100	0.396	0.394	0.305	0.304	0.398	0.397	0.307	0.306	0.534	0.529	0.489	0.484

tion as in Fig. 2.10 and asking for 500 replications of MDS analyses with random data, we would run `distrib <- randomstress(n = 40, ndim = 2, nrep = 500, type = "ordinal")` and then check the resulting distribution. For example, `mean(distrib)` delivers the mean value; `quantile(distrib, .05)` the 5th percentile and `min(distrib)` the smallest Stress value of any MDS in the simulation.

In practical applications, one almost always finds that the observed Stress value is clearly smaller than Stress values that can be expected for random data. For example, for the case in Fig. 2.10, Table 3.3 shows that the expected random Stress is 0.358, with a 5% of 0.353. The Stress value for the (ordinal) MDS solution in Fig. 2.10 is 0.179, and thus much smaller than these benchmark values. Indeed, it is even smaller than the minimal Stress value found in the `randomstress()` simulation (0.347).

To see how Stress depends more generally on the number of points, on the dimensionality of the MDS solution, and on the type of regression used by the MDS model, consider Fig. 3.2 (Mair et al. 2016). It shows that we can expect that more points, stronger scale-level assumptions (i.e., interval vs. ordinal), and smaller dimensionality lead to higher Stress values. In other words, the more restrictive the MDS model, the higher the Stress in general. The figure also shows that ordinal and interval MDS do not differ much in terms of Stress (for random data sampled from $U(0, 1)$), but ratio MDS is definitely more difficult to fit to such random data.

Using random data to obtain a Stress distribution under a null hypothesis means that we are drawing dissimilarities from a population over which we assume a distribution that does not necessarily reflect the data-generating process under question. A more modern way to create a stress-sampling distribution under the null hypothesis of misfit is running a *permutation test* (Mair et al. 2016). Here, the given data (not just any random data) are permuted and then subjected to MDS. This is repeated many times and the distribution of the resulting Stress values is analyzed. Obviously, the

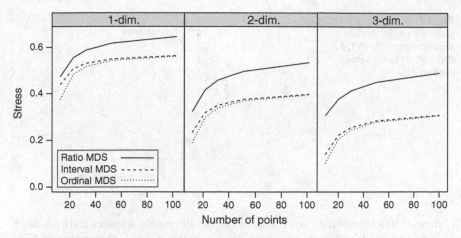

Fig. 3.2 Random Stress norms for ratio, interval, and ordinal MDS; for 1, 2, and 3 dimensions; and for different numbers of points (n)

outcome of such a test always depends on the particular data, and so no norm tables as in case of random data can be derived. However, when using SMACOF, a permutation test is easy. All the user has to do is run an MDS analysis (e.g., `my.results <- mds(dissim)`) and then evaluate the function `permtest(my.results)`. The program will generate and scale 100 data permutations and, in case of the country similarity data and the solution in Fig. 2.2, inform the user: `Observed stress value: 0.185 p-value: 0.03`. Hence, the Stress of 0.185 for these data is "significant" at the 5% level.[5] Note that the permutation test is somewhat stricter than the classical random Stress norms. It also takes into account basic properties of the given data. Therefore, it provides a sharper and more realistic null hypothesis than the one under fully random dissimilarities.

3.3 Stress and MDS Dimensionality

Increasing the dimensionality of the MDS space always makes it easier to find a solution with a better fit. Thus, Stress can be expected to drop as the dimensionality of the MDS space goes up. This is also evident from Fig. 3.2. The question we now ask is whether increasing the dimensionality of an MDS solution also leads to "significantly" smaller Stress values. To answer this question, one would first

---

[5]You can display this result graphically. For example, by `ex <- permtest(my.results); hist(ex$stressvec), xlim=c(ex$stress.obs-.05, max(ex$stressvec) +.05)); abline(v=ex$stress.obs, col="red"); points(ex$stress.obs, 0, cex = 2, pch = 16, col = "red")`. The plot shows the distribution of the Stress values for the permuted data, with a red vertical line at the point of the Stress value for the observed data.

Fig. 3.3 Scree plot of Stress
values of 1d–5d MDS
representations for PVQ40
data and for comparable
random data

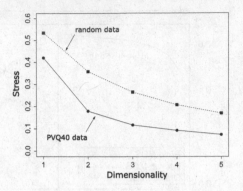

compute MDS solutions in, say, 1, 2, 3, and higher-dimensional spaces and then check
how the Stress values decrease when the dimensionality goes up. One way to evaluate
the effect is to compare the observed Stress values with Stress values for random data
and look for an elbow in the decreasing Stress versus Dimensionality function, similar
to scree tests in factor analysis. As simulation studies suggest (Spence and Graef
1974), the elbow indicates the dimensionality where additional dimensions represent
only random components of the data. In real (not simulated) data, however, elbows
are rarely pronounced. Consider such a plot for the personal value data discussed
above on p. 22. Figure 3.3 shows that the expected Stress values for random data with
40 points drop rather smoothly when increasing the dimensionality of the (ordinal)
MDS space. The Stress values for the PVQ40 data are all considerably smaller, and
they also show a slight elbow at 2 (or, less strongly, at 3) dimensions. This is nice
to know, because theoretical reasons and many previous studies also suggest a 2d
solution for these data.

3.4   Stress Per Point

Stress is a *global* measure of fit, an aggregation of all representation errors. A fit
index that lies between the global Stress and the individual representation errors is
the Stress contribution of a single point, called *Stress per Point* (SPP). It is computed
by first averaging the squared representation errors related to p. For example, for
the point Egypt we turn to Table 3.1 and sum the representation errors in row Egypt
(0.011, 0.000, 0.187) and in column Egypt (0.010, 0.013, ... , 0.029). This yields
0.046. We then express this value as the percentage of the sum of all representation
errors: $0.46/4.52 \cdot 100$. The contribution of Egypt to the total Stress is, therefore,
10.25%.

SPP values are automatically produced by SMACOF when running `result <-
mds(..)`. They can be called from the output object `result` by the command
`result$spp`:

Fig. 3.4 Bubble plot for
country similarity ratings;
size of bubble represents
SPP of country

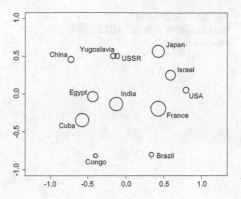

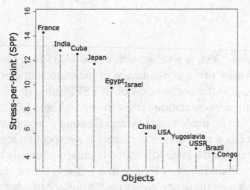

Fig. 3.5 SPP values for country similarity MDS solution in Fig. 2.2

Brazil	Congo	Cuba	Egypt	France	India	Israel	Japan	China	USSR	USA	Yugoslavia
4.19	3.51	12.27	10.25	14.35	13.29	9.75	11.38	5.71	4.70	5.49	5.11

The SPP values can be exhibited graphically within a normal MDS plot by drawing the points as bubbles (Fig. 3.4). There is also a function to plot the distribution of the SPP values: The command plot(result, plot.type = "stressplot") produces Fig. 3.5. It shows that there are no true outliers, but quite some scatter in terms of fit among the points. Why France is the highest Stress contributor and Congo the country with the relatively best fit, needs to be investigated by further research. One reason could be that France is a country that generates a relatively complex mental representation so that different respondents may use different criteria when comparing it to other countries. Congo, on the other hand, could be just the opposite: The respondents may all perceive it in the same way as a developing African country.

When assessing SPP values, one should first note that they become smaller the more points there are, because the SPP's are just contribution percentages of the total raw Stress. The mean value of the SPP's is always $100/n$ (%), with n the number of points. Moreover, with real and noisy data, there should always be some scatter

Fig. 3.6 Heatmap of
representation errors of MDS
solution in Fig. 2.2

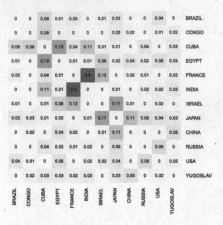

about this mean value.[6] Yet, is a value such as the 14.35 for France a substantively
meaningful deviation or just a consequence of measurement error? To answer this
question, we can look at the components of this SPP value in more detail, that is at
the distribution of the representation errors shown in Table 3.2 (lower half). Understanding this table can be made easier by representing it as a heat map as shown in
Fig. 3.6 where the cells are the darker the larger the respective representation error.[7]
For France, one notes that the large SPP value is caused primarily by one single comparison, the perceived similarity of France and India. It seems that the respondents
had problems to compare these two countries ("Similar? In what sense?").

3.5 Conditions Causing High Stress in MDS

Evaluating a given Stress value is a complex matter. It involves a number of different
parameters and considerations:

- The number of points (n): The greater n, the larger the expected Stress (because the
  number of distances in an MDS solution grows almost quadratically as a function
  of n).

---

[6]Simulations using pure random data show that in case of 12 points the SPP values scatter about
8.33 with an *sd* of 3.10; 96% of the SPPs are in the range from 14.53 to 2.13.

[7]This heat map is generated by `library(gplots); diss <-  sim2diss`
`(wish, method=7); res <-     mds(diss, type="ordinal"); RepErr <-`
`as.matrix((res$dhat - res$confdist)^2); yr <-     colorRampPalette`
`(c("lightyellow", "red"), space = "rgb")(100); heatmap.2( RepErr,`
`cellnote=round(RepErr,2), Rowv = NA, Colv = "Rowv", lhei=c(0.05,`
`0.15), margins = c(8, 8), key=FALSE, notecol = "black", trace =`
`"none", col = yr, symm = TRUE, dendrogram = "none")` , where RepErr is
the matrix of representation errors.

- The dimensionality of the MDS solution (m): The greater m, the smaller the expected Stress (because higher-dimensional spaces offer more freedom for an optimal positioning of points).
- The error component of the data: The greater the noise in the data, the larger the expected Stress (random data require maximal dimensionality).
- The MDS model: Stronger MDS models lead to higher Stress values than weaker MDS models, because they leave less freedom for choosing optimal $\widehat{d}_{ij}$ values.
- The number of ties when using the primary approach to ties in ordinal MDS (see Sect. 5.1): The more ties (=equal values) in the proximities, the smaller the expected Stress. The reason is that the primary approach to ties does not require that ties be mapped into equal distances, so MDS has more freedom to find an optimal solution.
- The proportion of missing proximities (missing data): The more data are missing, the easier it is to find an MDS solution with small Stress.
- Outliers and other special cases: Different points contribute differently to the total Stress; eliminating particular points or setting certain data as missing (e.g., because they are errors), can reduce the total Stress considerably.

3.6   Stress in Unfolding

Evaluating the fit of unfolding solutions is in principle the same as in MDS, but statistical benchmarks have not been published yet for unfolding. The user would have to either compute them him-/herself using random data in a cycle of unfolding analyses, or use the function `unfolding()` in SMACOF, because it offers a significance test. This test is a permutation test which is actually a sharper test than a test based on random data. If `result <- unfolding(..)` is given, then the test is simply called by `permtest(result)`. Moreover, `unfolding` also computes and plots SPP values for both row and column points (see example in Fig. 8.1).

3.7   Stability of MDS Solutions

An important issue when evaluating the goodness of an MDS solution is its stability. That is, does the configuration remain essentially the same if, for example, one of the points was removed? This question can be answered by jackknifing, a resampling technique that systematically leaves out one observation from the dataset and computes an MDS solution for the $n - 1$ remaining data (De Leeuw and Meulman 1986). Jackknifing is offered by SMACOF. Given the output object `result <- mds(..)`, you can call `JK <- jackknife(result)` to compute the jackknife. Then, simply typing `JK` gives you a "stability measure." This measure is hard to evaluate without benchmarks but `plot(JK)` exhibits the MDS configuration together with a star of

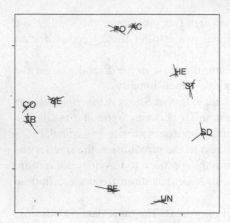

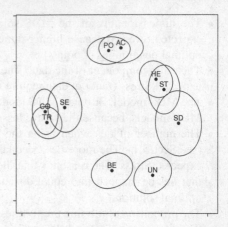

Fig. 3.7 Jackknife plot for personal values data; labels show MDS configuration; star shows jackknife stability

Fig. 3.8 Bootstrapping of MDS solution of personal values; ellipses indicate 95% confidence regions of points

lines attached to each point that gives you an impression of the stability of the MDS configuration under the various $n - 1$ conditions.

We show this in Fig. 3.7 for the ten personal value indexes and their MDS solution in Fig. 2.13. The end point of the stars show the respective point positions of the $n - 1$ jackknife configurations, fitted to each other, and subsequently connected to their centroid. We here see that this MDS configuration is almost not affected at all when single points are left out. That is true for any point.

More useful for the applied MDS user is bootstrapping (Jacoby and Armstrong 2014). It requires that you have a person-by-variable matrix from which the proximities are derived. If these proximities are the correlations of the columns, then the following code[8] gives you the interval MDS solution of Fig. 3.8 together with ellipses surrounding each point that represents a personal value PO, ... , SE (Fig. 3.8). These ellipses mark the 95% confidence regions of the points. They are reasonably compact, indicating that our ordinal MDS analysis has identified a configuration of points that are likely to lie at or close to the reported positions.

---

[8]Note that we first compute an MDS solution and then use the solution as the first argument when calling boot. The second argument is the data file; the third is the type of proximity measure for the variables; and the fourth is the number of bootstrapping samples you want the function to draw. It is set here to 500.

```
1  R <- cor(PVQ40agg); diss <- sim2diss(R)
2  result <- mds(diss, type="ordinal")  ## 2D ordinal MDS
3  set.seed(123)
4  resboot <- bootmds(result, data=PVQ40agg, method.dat="pearson", nrep=500)
5  plot(resboot, main="", xlab="", ylab="", col.axis = "white", ell=list(lty=1,
        col="black", cex=2, label.conf=list(label=TRUE, pos=3, col=1, cex=1.5)))
```

3.8 Summary

The formal goodness of an MDS solution is measured by computing the solution's
Stress. Stress is a loss function: It is zero if the solution is perfect; otherwise, it is
greater than zero. Stress aggregates the representation errors of each data-distance
pair. They correspond to the (vertical) deviations from the regression line in a data-
vs.-distances plot (Shepard diagram). When evaluating the Stress value of a particular
MDS solution, the user must assess it in the context of various parameters and con-
tingencies such as the number of points, the dimensionality of the MDS space, the
rigidity of the particular MDS model, and the reliability of the data. A minimum
criterion for an acceptably low Stress value is that it is clearly smaller than the Stress
expected for random data. It is often useful to also study the contributions of the
various variables of the data matrix to the global Stress (Stress per Point, SPP) and
even the single representation errors of any Stress measure. This may help identify
outliers and other reasons for high Stress. Stability is another criterion of goodness of an MDS solution. It can be evaluated using jackknifing and bootstrapping.
Bootstrapping generates confidence regions for the points of the MDS configuration.

References

Borg, I., & Groenen, P. J. F. (2005). *Modern Multidimensional Scaling* (2nd ed.). New York:
    Springer.
De Leeuw, J., & Meulman, J. (1986). A special jackknife for multidimensional scaling. *Journal of
    Classification, 3*, 97–112.
Jacoby, W. G., & Armstrong, D. A. (2014). Bootstrap confidence regions for multidimensional
    scaling solutions. *American Journal of Political Science, 58*, 264–278.
Mair, P., Borg, I., & Rusch, T. (2016). Goodness-of-fit assessment in multidimensional scaling and
    unfolding. *Multivariate Behavioral Research, 51*, 772–789.
Spence, I., & Graef, J. (1974). The determination of the underlying dimensionality of an empirically
    obtained matrix of proximities. *Multivariate Behavioral Research, 9*, 331–341.
Spence, I., & Ogilvie, J. C. (1973). A table of expected stress values for random rankings in
    nonmetric multidimensional scaling. *Multivariate Behavioral Research, 8*, 511–517.

Chapter 4
Proximities

Abstract The data for MDS, proximities, are discussed. Proximities can be collected directly as judgments of similarity; proximities can be derived from data vectors; proximities may result from converting other indexes; and co-occurrence data are yet another popular form of proximities.

Keywords Similarity ratings · Sorting method · Feature model · LCJ model
Co-occurrence data · S-coefficient · Jaccard coefficient · Simple matching
coefficient · Gravity model

A major advantage of MDS over related statistical methods (e.g., factor analysis) is that MDS can handle very different data as long as these data can be interpreted as proximities, i.e., as measures of similarity or dissimilarity. They can be collected either directly (e.g., as numerical ratings of similarity), or they can be derived from other data (e.g., correlations).

4.1 Direct Proximities

In Sect. 2.2, we discussed a study where the similarity of different countries was assessed by asking persons to rate the similarity of all pairs of 12 different countries on a rating scale. More concretely, each pair of countries (e.g., "Japan–China") was presented to the respondents, together with a rating scale with nine categories numbered from 1 to 9 and labeled as "very different" (for category 1) to "very similar" (for category 9). This method generated 66 pairwise ratings per person, enough data to scale each single person via MDS. A similar procedure was used in Sect. 2.3, where a sample of subjects was asked to judge the pairwise similarities of 16 different rectangles on a 10-point rating scale ranging from "0=equal, identical" to "9=very different."

Pairwise similarity ratings can become difficult for the respondents. The rating scale may be too fine-grained (or too coarse) for some respondents so that their ratings become unreliable. Market researchers, therefore, typically prefer a *sorting*

© The Author(s) 2018
I. Borg et al., *Applied Multidimensional Scaling and Unfolding*,
SpringerBriefs in Statistics, https://doi.org/10.1007/978-3-319-73471-2_4

method over ratings, where the subjects work with a deck of cards. Each card exhibits exactly one pair of objects (e.g., the pair "Japan–China"). The subjects are asked to sort the cards so that the card with the most similar pair is on top of the deck, and the card showing the most dissimilar pair at the bottom. Since a complete sorting of all cards is often time-consuming and difficult, the sorting is often simplified: The subjects are asked to begin by sorting the cards into only two stacks, one for the "similar" pairs, and one for the "dissimilar" pairs. For each stack, this two-stacks sorting is repeated several times until the subjects feel that they cannot reliably split the remaining stacks any further. One then numbers the various stacks from most similar to least similar pairs and assigns these numbers to the pairs in the respective stacks. Thus, pairs that belong to the same stack receive the same similarity score.

These examples show that collecting direct proximities can be done on the basis of relatively simple judgments. However, pairwise ratings and card sortings also have their drawbacks. They can both lead to an excessively large number of pairs that must be judged by the subjects. For the $n = 12$ countries of the study in Sect. 2.2, for example, each subject had to rate 66 different pairs of countries. That seems acceptable, but for $n = 20$ countries, say, the number of different pairs goes up to $n \cdot (n - 1)/2 = 190$. Assessing that many pairs (even without replications) is a challenge even for a very motivated test person. To alleviate this problem, various designs for reducing the number of pair comparisons have been developed. It was found that a random sample of all possible pairs is not only a simple but also a good method of reduction: One collects only data on the pairs that belong to the random sample and sets the proximities of all other pairs to "missing" (NA).

Spence and Domoney (1974) showed in extensive simulation studies that the proportion of missing data can be as high as 80% and (ordinal) MDS is still able to recover an underlying MDS configuration quite precisely. One should realize, however, that these simulations made a number of simplifying assumptions that cannot automatically be taken for granted in real applications. The simulations first defined some random configuration in m-dimensional space. The distances among its points were then superimposed with random noise and taken as proximities. Finally, certain proximities were eliminated either randomly or per systematic design. The m-dimensional MDS configurations computed from these data were then compared with the m-dimensional configurations that served to generate the data. The precision with which MDS was able to reconstruct the original configurations from the proximities was found to depend on the proportion of missing data; on the proportion of random noise superimposed onto the distances; and on the number of points. In all simulated cases, the dimensionality of the MDS solution was equal to the true dimensionality, and the number of points was relatively large from an MDS user's point of view (i.e., 32 or more). Under these conditions, MDS was able to tolerate large proportions of missing data. If, for example, one-third of the proximities is missing and the error component is equal to 15%, then the MDS distances can be expected to correlate with $r = 0.97$ with the original distances!

One can improve the robustness of MDS by collecting primarily proximities of pairs of objects that seem very dissimilar rather than similar, because one thus has proximities for the large distances and they are particularly important for the precision of recovery (Graef and Spence 1979).

The labor involved in data collection can be further reduced by simplifying the individual similarity judgments. Rather than asking for graded ratings on, say, a 10-point scale, one may offer only two response categories, "similar" (1) and "dissimilar" (0) for each pair of objects. Summing such dichotomous data over replications or over respondents leads to confusion frequencies or, after dividing by the number of cases, to confusion probabilities. Yet, such aggregations are not necessarily required. Green and Wind (1973) showed in a simulation study that robust MDS is possible using coarse data—given advantageous side constraints such as scaling in the true dimensionality and having many points. The study shows, though, that *some* grading of the data is better than 1-0 data, but very fine grading has essentially no effect on the robustness of MDS. Hence, if one collects direct proximities, it is not necessary to measure up to many decimals (if that is possible at all); rather, nine or ten scale categories are sufficient for MDS.

4.2   Derived Proximities

Direct proximities are rather rare in practice. Most applications of MDS are based on proximity indexes derived from pairs of data vectors. One example is the proximities used in Chap. 1, where the correlations of the frequencies of different crimes in different states were taken as proximities of these crimes.

Indexes of similarity are often used in market research. Assume we want to assess the subjective similarity of different cars. Proximities could be generated by first asking a sample of test persons to rate the cars we are interested in on such attributes as design, fuel consumption, price, and performance. Then, the correlations of the ratings for each pair of cars can be taken as an indicator of their perceived similarity.

Instead of using correlation coefficients, one can also consider measuring the similarity of data profiles by the Euclidean or by the city-block distance. Such distances can differ substantially from correlations. If, for example, two variables with n elements each have the same profile of ups and downs so that their values differ by an additive constant a only, their correlation is $r = 1$ and their Euclidean distance is $a\sqrt{n}$. Conversely, two variables with distance $a\sqrt{n}$ correlate with $r = -1$ if their profiles cross each other in the form of an X. Hence, whether one wants to use a correlation or a distance for measuring the proximity of profiles must be carefully considered.

If the variables are (im- or explicitly) standardized, the relation of correlations and (Euclidean) distances becomes simpler. Assume you have two variables, X and Y, both standardized so that they have zero means and sums-of-squares equal to 1. Their product-moment correlation is simply $r_{XY} = \sum_i x_i y_i$. Then, their Euclidean distance is

$$d_{XY} = \left(\sum_{i=1}^{N} (x_i - y_i)^2 \right)^{1/2}$$

$$= \left(\sum x_i^2 + \sum y_i^2 - 2 \sum x_i y_i \right)^{1/2}$$

$$= const \cdot \sqrt{(1 - r_{XY})}, \text{ where } const = \sqrt{2}. \qquad (4.1)$$

Hence, when using ordinal MDS, it becomes irrelevant which proximity measure is used, because both yield (inversely) *equivalent* rank orders. For interval MDS, using correlations or Euclidean distances also does not make much difference, because the two measures are almost linearly related.[1]

Besides Euclidean and other Minkowski distances, many other distance functions are used in data analysis. An interesting case is discussed by Restle (1959). In his feature models of similarity, he defines the distance between two psychological objects as the relative proportion of the elements in their mental representations that are specific for each object. That is, for example, if a person associates with Japan the features X, Y, and Z, and with China A, B, X, and Z, then their psychological distance is $3/5 = 0.6$, because there is a total of five different mental elements and three of them (Y, A, and B) are specific ones.

4.3   Proximities from Index Conversions

Proximities can sometimes be generated by theory-guided conversions of given measurements on pairs of objects. Here is one example. Glushko (1975) was interested in assessing the "psychological goodness" of dot patterns. He constructed a set of different patterns and printed each pair on a separate card. Twenty subjects were then asked to indicate which pattern in each pair is the "better" one. The pattern judged "better" received a score of 1, the other one a 0. These scores were summed over all subjects. A dissimilarity measure was constructed from these sums by subtracting 10 (i.e., the expected value for each pair of patterns if all 20 subjects would decide their preferences randomly) from each sum and then taking the absolute value of this difference.

Borg (1988) used a different conversion to turn dominance probabilities into proximities. In the older psychological literature, many data sets are reported where N persons are asked to judge which object in a pair of objects possesses more of a certain property. For example, considering crimes, the persons decide whether Murder is "more serious" than arson or not. Or, for paintings, is picture A "prettier" than

---

[1]For other forms of standardization, the results are essentially the same. For example, when turning the variables first into z-scores (with mean zero and $sd = 1$), Eq. (4.1) changes to $const = \sqrt{2N}$. Note, however, that when you compute a product-moment correlation, you implicitly standardize your variables. If that makes sense, you should also standardize them before computing distances, but then using correlations or distances does not make a difference in ordinal MDS.

picture B? The object chosen by the subjects receives a score of 1; the other object is rated as 0. If one then adds these dominance scores over all N subjects and divides by N, dominance probabilities, p_{ij}, are generated. Such data are often scaled by using Thurstone's law of comparative judgment procedure (Thurstone 1927). It assumes that each p_{ij} is related to the distance d_{ij} on a one-dimensional scale by a cumulative normal function. This rather strong assumption can be replaced by a weaker model that gives the data more room to speak for themselves: This model simply postulates that the dominance probabilities are related to distances by a monotonically increasing function, without specifying the exact form of this function. To find the function that best satisfies this model, ordinal MDS can be used. First, however, one needs to convert the dominance probabilities into dissimilarities via $\delta_{ij} = |p_{ij} - 0.5|$. Then, the MDS distances—negatively signed if $p_{ij} > 0.5$, meaning you have to move to the left from point i to get to j—are plotted against the p_{ij} probabilities. If Thurstone's model is correct, the regression trend should form an inverted S-shaped function running from the upper left-hand side to the lower right-hand side.

More examples for index conversions are discussed in Borg and Groenen (2005). We do not pursue this topic here further, because the two examples above should have made clear that it makes no sense to report such conversions one after the other in statistical textbooks. Rather, they always require substantive-theoretical considerations that can be quite specific for the particular setting.

4.4 Co-occurrence Data

An interesting special case of proximities are co-occurrence data. Here is one example. Coxon and Jones (1978) studied the categories that people use to classify occupations. Their subjects were asked to sort a set of 32 occupational titles (such as barman, statistician, and actor) on the basis of their overall similarity into as many or as few groups as they wished. The result of this sorting can be expressed, for each subject, by a 32×32 *incidence matrix*, $\mathbf{Z}$, with a score of 1 wherever its row and columns entries are sorted into the same group and 0 elsewhere.

The incidence matrix $\mathbf{Z}$ in the example above is a data matrix of directly collected same–different proximities. This is not always true for co-occurrence data, as the following study by England and Ruiz-Quintanilla (1994) demonstrates. These authors studied "the meaning of working." For that purpose, they asked large samples of persons to consider a variety of statements such as "if it is physically strenuous" or "if you have to do it" and check those statements that would define work for them. The similarity of two statements was then defined as the frequency with which they were both checked by the respondents. Note that "similarity" was never assessed directly. Rather, it was defined by the researchers. No person in these surveys was ever asked to directly judge the "similarity" or the "difference" of anything.

Co-occurrence data often consist of a binary presence–absence matrix. An example is a data matrix where the columns represent medical diseases, the rows different symptoms, and the entries the presence (1) or absence (0) of the symptom. For such

Table 4.1 Cumulative frequencies of co-occurrence types for column variables x and y across all rows; 1 and 0 indicate presence and absence, respectively, in the data matrix

	$x = 1$	$x = 0$	Sum
$y = 1$	a	b	$a + b$
$y = 0$	c	d	$c + d$
Sum	$a + c$	$b + d$	$a + b + c + d$

data, one can define surprisingly many similarity measures. For each pair of column variables x and y, there are four possible types of co-occurrence for each row variable: The row variable is present in both x and y (11); it is absent in both x and y (00); or it is present in one case but not in the other case (10 or 01). The observed frequencies of these types of co-occurrence for x and y across all rows of the data matrix are denoted as a, d, b, and c, respectively, as shown in Table 4.1.

Based on these frequencies, Gower (1985) proposed a system of similarity coefficients. One of them is

$$S_2 = a/(a + b + c + d) ,$$

the frequency of hits in both x and y, relative to the frequency of all possible combinations of hits in x and y ($= a + b + c + d$). Another coefficient is

$$S_3 = a/(a + b + c) ,$$

the frequency of joint occurrences in x and y, relative to the frequency of cases where at least one row variable is present in x and y (*Jaccard similarity index*).

Choosing a particular S-index over another such index can have dramatic consequences. Bilsky et al. (1994) report a study on different behaviors exhibited in family conflicts, ranging from calm discussions to physical assault. The intention was to find out in which psychologically meaningful ways such behaviors can be scaled. They conducted a survey asking which of a list of different conflict behaviors had occurred in the respondent's family in the last five years. If one assesses[2] the similarities of the reported behaviors by S_3, a subsequent MDS generates a one-dimensional scale on which the behaviors are arrayed from low to high aggression. This order makes psychological sense. If one uses S_2, however, then this simple solution falls apart. The reason is that the very aggressive behaviors are also relatively rare, which inflates d so that these behaviors become highly dissimilar in the S_2 sense.

Of the many further variants of S-coefficients (Gower 1985; Cox et al. 2000; Borg and Groenen 2005), we here mention the *simple matching coefficient*,

---

[2] An R-function, `dist.binary()`, for computing ten different S-coefficients—including S_2, S_3, and S_4 – among the columns of a binary data matrix can be found at https://rdrr.io/rforge/ade4/src/R/dist.binary.R.

$$S_4 = (a + d)/(a + b + c + d) \, ,$$

which interprets both the joint occurrence and the joint nonoccurrence of events as
a sign of similarity. In the above example of conflict behaviors, S_4 would assess the
rare forms of behavior as similar because they are rare.

4.5   The Gravity Model for Co-occurrences

Co-occurrences are, by themselves, almost never reasonable measures of similarity. Rather, they have to be expressed relative to other observed (or theoretically
expected) co-occurrences or occurrences—as shown above for the S-coefficients.
Another interesting approach to process co-occurrence data is the gravity model
which formulates a congruence coefficient for co-occurrence data that is directly
related to distance estimates.

Let c_{kk} denote the frequency with which stimulus k occurred in a given context,
and c_{ij} the frequency with which stimulus i and stimulus j co-occurred. Then, the
gravity model defines the dissimilarity of i and j as

$$\delta_{ij} = \left(\frac{c_{ii} c_{jj}}{c_{ij}} \right)^{1/2}, \quad \text{for} \quad c_{ij} > 0 \, . \tag{4.2}$$

In (4.2), $1/c_{ij}$ transforms the similarity measure c_{ij} into a dissimilarity score;
multiplying by $c_{ii} c_{jj}$ expresses the similarity relative to the product of the occurrences
of i and j; and the square root follows from the origin of the model in physics.

The gravity model is based on Newton's law of gravitation that expresses the
gravitational force F of two bodies with masses m_1 and m_2 and distance d as $F =
G \cdot (m_1 \cdot m_2)/d^2$, with G the gravitation constant. So, if we interpret F as the force
of mutual attraction of two observed stimuli ij, their co-occurrence c_{ij} as a measure
of that force, and the mass m_k as c_{kk}, we can estimate d as in formula (4.2).

Formula (4.2) leaves open what to do if two stimuli do not co-occur, that is, if
$c_{ij} = 0$. Obviously, in that case, we cannot compute δ_{ij} by this formula. Rather, we
need a reasonable definition. One solution is setting δ_{ij} equal to a number greater
than any dissimilarity based on nonzero co-occurrence data. This would not affect an
ordinal MDS (with the primary approach to ties) of the resulting dissimilarities, but
it would affect an interval MDS, for example. Thus, the preferred solution that works
for any type of MDS is defining δ_{ij} as missing ($=$NA) in the zero co-occurrence case
so that these values are skipped in MDS.[3]

Tobler and Wineburg (1971) used the gravity model and MDS in an intrigu-
ing application constructing a map of Assyrian merchant colonies in Bronze Age

---

[3]If you have many cases of no co-occurrence, then your dissimilarity matrix becomes very sparse.
Then, of course, MDS may become rather arbitrary, producing fancy configurations based on almost
no data.

Anatolia (Turkey) on the basis of data provided by the Cappadocian cuneiform tablets. They first formulated the gravity model as $I_{ij} = kP_iP_j/d_{ij}^2$, where "$I_{ij}$ is the interaction between places i and j; k is a constant, depending on the phenomena; P_i is the population of i; P_j is the population of j; and d_{ij} is the distance between places i and j. Distance may be in hours, dollars, or kilometers; populations may be in income, numbers of people, numbers of telephones, and so on; and the interaction may be in numbers of letters exchanged, number of marriages, similarity of artifacts or cultural traits, and so on" (p. 2). Tobler and Wineburg (1971) then chose the number of occurrences of a town's name on the cuneiform tablets as P_i, and the number of co-occurrences on the tablets as I_{ij}. The resulting distance estimates were used as input for a 2d ordinal MDS in an effort to find the (largely unknown) geographical map of the 62 "more important" places of 119 towns mentioned on the tablets.

Mair et al. (2014) report another application of the gravity model. They studied the semantic space of certain self-reported statements of Republican voters in the USA. These voters were asked to complete the sentence "I'am Republican, because ...". Their responses are published on the official Web site of the Republican party. 252 unique statements and the 35 most frequent key words were identified by text analysis methods. They were used to form a 252×35 incidence matrix $\mathbf{Z}$ with cells of 1 if statement i contains word j, and zero if not. The matrix product $\mathbf{Z}'\mathbf{Z}$ is the co-occurrence matrix $\mathbf{C}$ in formula (4.2).

$\mathbf{C}$ was then turned into dissimilarities using a slight extension of the above gravity model, the *power gravity model*. This model replaces the exponent 1/2 in formula (4.2) by $\lambda/2$. The exponent λ is chosen to weight the dissimilarities. With large exponents, large dissimilarities become relatively more important; with $\lambda = 1$, we get the simple gravity model; and with negative λ's, the impact of small dissimilarities on the MDS solution is increased. Mair et al. (2014) used $\lambda = 2$ for their data and remark that "there is a trade-off between the structure determined by λ and the goodness-of-fit as quantified by the Stress value: The more structure we create, the higher the Stress value" (p. 5). This is so because heavily weighting large dissimilarities, for example, makes it generally easier to find a low-Stress solution, because then most of the smaller dissimilarities have essentially zero weights in the Stress measure. With huge λ's, only very few dissimilarities matter.

In SMACOF, one can simply use the `gravity()` function to process the incidence matrix $\mathbf{Y}$ in the sense of the power gravity model. This makes it easy to use the model:

```
data(GOPdtm)
gravD <- gravity(GOPdtm, lambda = 2)
res <- mds(gravD$gravdiss)
res$weightmat ## NA's were blanked out when fitting the model
plot(res)
```

4.6 Summary

MDS builds on proximity data. Many data qualify as proximity data. In psychological research, proximities are sometimes collected directly by asking persons to
rate the perceived similarity of objects of interest on a numerical rating scale. A
convenient alternative is sorting a stack of cards, with one card per object pair, in
terms of the objects' similarity. Proximities can also be derived from other measures.
The inter-correlations of the variables in a typical person-by-variables data matrix,
for example, is a popular example. Sometimes, proximities can be constructed by
converting other measures on pairs of objects such as probabilities with which object
i dominates object j. Yet another form of proximity data are measures that build on
co-occurrence data, where the frequencies with which the events i and j, respectively,
occur or do not occur at time t are combined into an index of co-occurrence such as
Gower's S-indexes or the Jaccard index. For co-occurrence data with very skewed
distributions, the gravity model offers one possibility to generate dissimilarities that
lead to meaningful MDS solutions.

References

Bilsky, W., Borg, I., & Wetzels, P. (1994). Assessing connfict tactics in close relationships: A
    reanlysis of a research instrument. In J. J. Hox, P. G. Swanborn, & G. J. Mellenbergh (Eds.),
    Facet theory: Analysis and design (pp. 39–46). Zeist, The Netherlands: Setos.
Borg, I. (1988). Revisiting Thurstone's and Coombs' scales on the seriousness of crimes and
    offences. *European Journal of Social Psychology, 18*, 53–61.
Borg, I., & Groenen, P. J. F. (2005). *Modern multidimensional scaling* (2nd ed.). New York: Springer.
Cox, T. F., & Cox, M. A. A. (2000). *Multidimensional scaling* (2nd ed.). London: Chapman & Hall.
Coxon, A. P. M., & Jones, C. L. (1978). *The images of occupational prestige: A study in social
    cognition.* London: Macmillan.
England, G., & Ruiz-Quintanilla, S. A. (1994). How working is defined: Structure and stability.
    In I. Borg & S. Dolan (Eds.), Proceedings of the Fourth International Conference on Work and
    Organizational Values (pp. 104–113). Montreal: ISSWOV.
Glushko, R. J. (1975). Pattern goodness and redundancy revisited: Multidimensional scaling and
    hierarchical clustering analyses. *Perception & Psychophysics, 17*, 158–162.
Gower, J. C. (1985). Measures of similarity, dissimilarity, and distance. In S. Kotz, N. L. Johnson,
    & C. B. Read (Eds.), Encyclopedia of statistical sciences (Vol. 5, pp. 397–405). New York: Wiley.
Graef, J., & Spence, I. (1979). Using distance information in the design of large multidimensional
    scaling experiments. *Psychological Bulletin, 86*, 60–66.
Green, P. E., & Wind, Y. (1973). *Multivariate decisions in marketing: A measurement approach.*
    Hinsdale, IL: Dryden.
Mair, P., Rusch, T., & Hornik, K. (2014). The grand old party: A party of values? *SpringerPlus,
    3*(697), 1–10.
Restle, F. (1959). A metric and an ordering on sets. *Psychometrika, 24*, 207–220.
Spence, I., & Domoney, D. W. (1974). Single subject incomplete designs for nonmetric multidi-
    mensional scaling. *Psychometrika, 39*, 469–490.
Thurstone, L. L. (1927). A law of comparative judgment. *Psychological Review, 34*, 273–286.
Tobler, W., & Wineburg, S. (1971). A cappadocian speculation. *Nature, 231*, 39–41.

Chapter 5
Variants of MDS Models

Abstract Various forms of MDS are discussed: ordinal MDS, metric MDS, MDS with different distance functions, MDS for asymmetric proximities, individual difference MDS models, MDS for more than one proximity value per distance, and weighting proximities in MDS.

Keywords Ordinal MDS · Interval MDS · Ratio MDS · Drift vector model
INDSCAL · IDIOSCAL · Unfolding

5.1 The Type of Regression in MDS

A main difference of various MDS models is the type of regression that these models use. The most popular MDS model in research publications has been *ordinal* MDS, sometimes also—less precisely—called *nonmetric* MDS. Ordinal MDS computes an m-dimensional configuration $\mathbf{X}$ so that the order of the distances over $\mathbf{X}$ deviates as little as possible from the order of the proximities. Hence, in ordinal MDS and assuming that we have dissimilarities δ_{ij} as data (or that the proximities have been converted into dissimilarities), the representation function

$$f : \delta_{ij} \rightarrow d_{ij}(\mathbf{X}) \qquad (5.1)$$

is *monotone* so that

$$f : \delta_{ij} < \delta_{kl} \rightarrow d_{ij}(\mathbf{X}) \leq d_{kl}(\mathbf{X}) \qquad (5.2)$$

for all pairs i and j, and k and l, respectively, for which data (dissimilarities) are given. Proximities that are not defined ("missing data") are skipped. That is, if p_{ij} is missing, it imposes no restriction onto the MDS solution so that the distance $d_{ij}(\mathbf{X})$ can be chosen arbitrarily.

An important distinction between two forms of ordinal MDS is how *ties* (i.e., equal data values) are treated. The default in most programs is that ties can be *broken* in the MDS solution. That means that equal proximities need *not* be mapped into

© The Author(s) 2018
I. Borg et al., *Applied Multidimensional Scaling and Unfolding*,
SpringerBriefs in Statistics, https://doi.org/10.1007/978-3-319-73471-2_5

equal distances. This is called the *primary approach to ties*. The *secondary* approach to ties ("keep ties tied") leads to an additional requirement for ordinal MDS, namely

$$f : \delta_{ij} = \delta_{kl} \rightarrow d_{ij}(\mathbf{X}) = d_{kl}(\mathbf{X}). \tag{5.3}$$

The primary approach to ties is usually more meaningful. Consider, for example, the data discussed in Sect. 2.2 where subjects had to judge the similarity of different countries on 9-point rating scales. Here, ties are unavoidable, because the rating scale had only nine different levels: With 66 different pairs of countries, this will automatically lead to the same proximity values for some pairs, even if the respondent feels that the respective countries are not really equally similar. Using a 66-point rating scale would not help either, because no respondent can make reliable distinctions on such a scale. Moreover, each single judgment is somewhat fuzzy and not absolutely reliable. Hence, equal ratings often mean something like "about equal" or "practically equal" but not simply "equal."

A second class of MDS models, called *metric* MDS, goes back to the beginnings of MDS in the 1950's (Torgerson 1952). Such models specify an analytic (usually monotone) function for f rather than requiring that f must be only "some" monotone function. Specifying analytic mapping functions for f has the advantage that it becomes easier to trace the mathematical properties of such models. Moreover, metric MDS avoids some technical problems of ordinal MDS such as, in particular, degenerate solutions (see Sect. 7.5). On the other hand, they typically lead to solutions with poorer fit to the data, because it is generally more difficult to represent data in more restrictive models. Yet, this may not be a drawback, because an excellent fit can also mean that more error is represented in the MDS solution. Ordinal MDS tends to over-fit the data, while metric MDS may iron out error in the data so that the solution becomes more robust and replicable.

The standard model of metric MDS is *interval MDS*, where

$$f : \delta_{ij} \rightarrow a + b \cdot \delta_{ij} = d_{ij}(\mathbf{X}), \tag{5.4}$$

with a and b ($\neq 0$) as free parameters. Interval MDS attempts to preserve the data in the distances such that the relations of *differences* ("intervals") among the data are preserved.[1] This makes sense, for example, if the data are interval-scaled. In that case, no meaningful information is lost if the data are scaled by multiplying them by some nonzero constant b and by adding an arbitrary constant a to each data value. All statements about the data that remain invariant under such linear transformations are considered meaningful; all other statements (e.g., statements about the ratio of data values) are not meaningful.

---

[1]Consider Table 1.1. Auto Theft and Murder are correlated with .11; Rape and Larceny with .60; the difference between these correlations is .49. This is about the same as the correlation between Assault and Burglary (.52). So, in the interval MDS solution in Fig. 1.4, the difference of the distances between the points for Auto Theft and for Murder should be about equal to the distance between Assault and Burglary.

More MDS models follow easily by choosing other mapping functions f (e.g., an exponential or a power function). However, if f is not at least weakly monotone, then such functions do not lead to easily interpretable results.

An MDS model that is stronger than interval MDS is *ratio MDS*, often considered the most restrictive model in MDS. It drops the additive constant a of interval MDS as an admissible transformation and searches for a solution that preserves the proximities up to an overall scaling factor b ($b \neq 0$). In case of the rectangle data analyzed in Chap. 2, this model could be seriously considered, because here the response scale started at "0=equal, identical" and hence scores of zero are meaningful if the subjects used the scale correctly.

The user chooses a particular MDS model f for a variety of reasons:

- Scale level. If theoretical or empirical reasons speak for a certain scale level of the data, then it usually makes sense to pick a corresponding MDS model. The choice of an appropriate scale level also depends on the zeitgeist to some extent. In the 1970s, for example, ordinal MDS was heavily pushed, whereas today metric (even: ratio) MDS has become the default (at least for statisticians) since it forces the user to justify any substantively blind optimizing transformations of the data.
- Minimize assumptions. The researcher wants to assume as little as possible about the relation of the data to MDS distances. Rather, he/she wants to let the data speak for themselves. Or he/she wants to get something for as little as possible. A typical case is a small inter-correlation matrix that is scaled with ordinal MDS and then interpreted in terms of dimensions or in terms of regions with wildly curving boundaries and many misplaced points. This can be useful as a first step in a field of research where little is known, but, of course, it should be replaced with more restrictive models in the long run.
- Robustness versus over-fitting. One often scales given proximities with both ordinal MDS and interval MDS. Ordinal MDS leads to smaller Stress values than interval MDS, but it may simply over-fit the data and, occasionally, it can also lead to meaningless degenerate solutions (see Sect. 7.5). Hence, when running both ordinal MDS and interval MDS, one can cross-validate the solutions and test for artifacts.
- Nonlinear mappings. The proximities are sometimes predicted to have a nonlinear relation to the distances in an MDS space. One example is Thurstone scaling, discussed on p. 47. In that case, one may not know how to specify the regression function analytically, or no program exists that would fit such a model, or one may want to test a certain prediction about the regression trend but not enforce it. So, ordinal MDS is used and then the Shepard diagram is studied closely for the shape of the regression trend. One may also first replace the data with their ranks and then use interval MDS: Weeks and Bentler (1979) have shown in simulations that this *rank-linear MDS* successfully recovers configurations whose distances have highly nonlinear (but still monotone) relations to the data.
- Dimensionality. Using weak MDS models leads to relatively small Stress values. This is often taken as evidence that one does not need higher-dimensional representation spaces. After all, if the Stress is small, then there is little left to explain.

This reasoning is somewhat too formal, though, because what one is really interested in are meaningful and replicable solutions. The Stress of the solution is but a technical index.

• Marketing. The user wants to get a small Stress value, because he/she fears that otherwise his/her results will not be publishable. This is, of course, a poor reason, because the Stress must always be evaluated relative to the particular MDS model, the dimensionality of the solution space, the number of points, and many other criteria such a robustness, stability, and replicability (Mair et al. 2016).

MDS models with other regression functions than those based on Steven's four classical scale levels exist too. One example is MDS with *spline transformations* on the data. Splines are piecewise (connected in k knots) polynomial functions of the n-th degree that lead to smooth (but not necessarily linear or monotone) regression lines in Shepard diagrams. The knots and the degree of the polynomials control the spline.

To illustrate what happens when running different types of MDS with real data, we use the inter-correlations in Table 2.2. Figure 5.1 exhibits the Shepard diagrams of 2d MDS solutions for these correlations. They show that ratio MDS fails completely, not because the regression trend is not nearly linear, but because the regression line must run through the origin: Only then are the data mapped into distances that preserve their ratios. The spline regression here is forced to run through the origin too. It is almost completely linear and has almost the same Stress as interval MDS.

Figure 5.1 shows, moreover, that ordinal MDS and interval MDS arrive at similar conclusions. The regression trend in ordinal MDS is almost linear, except for local steps and dents that are not interpretable and most likely not replicable. Yet, the Stress for ordinal MDS is clearly smaller than the Stress for interval MDS, simply because the regression line is closer to the points in the Shepard diagram in case of ordinal

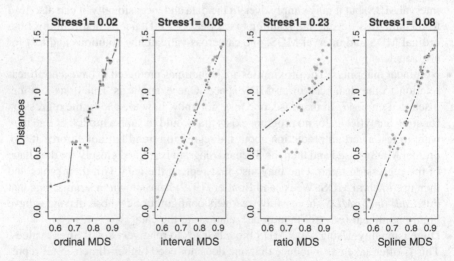

Fig. 5.1 Shepard diagrams for four types of regression; data from Table 2.4

MDS. Experience with empirical data shows that ordinal MDS and interval MDS often lead to highly similar results. Simulation studies come to the same conclusion (see Fig. 3.2). Ratio MDS is typically found to be much more demanding than either ordinal or interval MDS.

5.2   Euclidean and Other Distances

A second criterion for classifying MDS models is choosing a particular distance function. In psychology, the family of Minkowski metrics (specified in formula 2.3) used to be popular for modeling subjective similarity judgments of different types of stimuli (analyzable vs. integral stimuli) under different conditions (such as time, pressure). However, applications of MDS in the current literature almost always use Euclidean distances, because only they guarantee that the geometry is not misleading. Few MDS programs are even able to compute solutions with distances other than Euclidean distances. If they offer other distance functions too, then typically only the city-block metric.

Euclidean distances, as all other Minkowski distances, imply a *flat* geometry. In special cases, it can be useful to construct MDS representations in *curved* spaces. As an example, one can think of distances on a sphere. Here, the distance between two points is the shortest path ("geodesic path") in the two-dimensional curved space (i.e., on the sphere), which is the length of a cord spanned between two points over the surface of the sphere or, expressed more sloppily, airline distances. Curved geometries can sometimes be useful (e.g., in psychophysics), but they are never used in general data analysis situations. Circular scales do, however, play an important role in psychology, but they do not require true curved-space analysis. Rather, they use circles or balls embedded in Euclidean spaces. See, for example, "spherical MDS" on p. 72 and "circular unfolding" on p. 103.

5.3   MDS of Asymmetric Proximities

Distances are always symmetric, i.e., $d_{ij} = d_{ji}$, for all i, j. Proximities that are not symmetric can, therefore, not be represented by distances in MDS models. Yet, as long as the asymmetries are just error-based, no real problem arises. MDS simply irons out these errors. Or the user eliminates or reduces them by averaging corresponding data values.

Asymmetries may, however, be reliable and meaningful. Examples are the asymmetries in an import–export matrix, where country i imports more from county j than vice versa. Then, social networks can be studied in terms of how much each person i likes the other person j: Liking is rarely fully symmetric, and asymmetries can be very meaningful. A third example is simply the order of presentation when making pairwise comparisons of i and j: How similar is the Morse code di-di-da to the subsequent da-di, and how similar is da-di to the following di-di-da (see p. 70)?

A simple approach of dealing with asymmetric proximities in the MDS context is the *drift vector model*. The model requires decomposing the proximity matrix $\mathbf{P}$ into a symmetric part $\mathbf{S}$ and an asymmetric part $\mathbf{A}$. The symmetric part is computed by averaging corresponding cells, $\mathbf{S} = (\mathbf{P} + \mathbf{P}')/2$, with elements $s_{ij} = (p_{ij} + p_{ji})/2$. This matrix is then scaled as usual with MDS. The rest of the proximities is $\mathbf{A} = \mathbf{P} - \mathbf{S}$, with elements $a_{ij} = p_{ij} - s_{ij}$. This matrix is *skew-symmetric*. It can be represented on top of the MDS solution for $\mathbf{S}$ by attaching an arrow on each point i that is directed toward point j, or away from point j, depending on the sign of the asymmetry. The length of this arrow is chosen as $k \cdot |a_{ij}|$, with k some convenient overall scaling factor (e.g., $k = 1/\mathrm{mean}(p_{ij})$).

We demonstrate this model with a small example. Let $\mathbf{P}$ be a matrix of similarity values (e.g., the number of references in row journal i to column journal j):

$$\mathbf{P} = \begin{bmatrix} 0 & 4 & 6 & 13 \\ 5 & 0 & 37 & 21 \\ 4 & 38 & 0 & 16 \\ 8 & 31 & 18 & 0 \end{bmatrix} = \mathbf{S} + \mathbf{A} = \begin{bmatrix} 0 & 4.5 & 5.0 & 10.5 \\ 4.5 & 0 & 37.5 & 26.0 \\ 5.0 & 37.5 & 0 & 17.0 \\ 10.5 & 26.0 & 17.0 & 0 \end{bmatrix} + \begin{bmatrix} 0.0 & -0.5 & 1.0 & 2.5 \\ 0.5 & 0.0 & -0.5 & -5.0 \\ -1.0 & 0.5 & 0.0 & -1.0 \\ -2.5 & 5.0 & 1.0 & 0.0 \end{bmatrix}.$$

For $\mathbf{S}$, interval MDS yields the point configuration in Fig. 5.2. The values of $\mathbf{A}$ are represented as arrows in this plot. They are inserted one by one into the MDS solution. For example, on point #2, an arrow with a length of 5 units is attached pointing toward point #4. The resultant of all arrows attached to a point is the *drift vector* of that point, represented by the thick arrows with larger arrow heads in Fig. 5.2.

One notices in this vector field that, for example, journals #2 and #3 refer to each other relatively often and also quite symmetrically (because these points are close, and because the drift vectors are short). For journals #2 and #4, the mutual referencing is clearly smaller and, moreover, it is also rather asymmetric: Journal #2 looks more toward #4 than vice versa.

One can experiment somewhat with how one wants to represent the symmetries and the asymmetries (e.g., show all arrows or only resultant vectors; only vectors with the same meaning; use different scale factors for lengths of arrows). This can easily be done by using and modifying the R script for plotting Fig. 5.2 in the supplementary code file.

Let us look at a real data example. Rothkopf (1957) studied to what extent 598 test persons confused different acoustic Morse signals. He used 36 different signals, the 26 letters of the alphabet, and the natural numbers from 0 to 9. In the experiment, each person had to judge whether two signals, i and j, presented acoustically one after the other, were the same or not the same. Both (i, j) and (j, i) had to be judged in the experiment. The percentage of "Same!" judgments (i.e., the confusion probability) for each pair is taken as a measure of the psychological similarity of each pair.

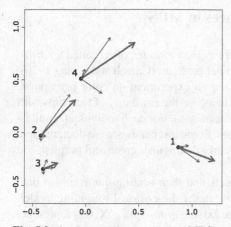

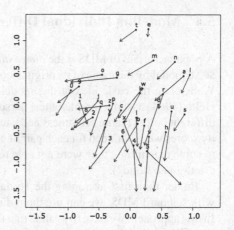

Fig. 5.2 Asymmetry vectors over an MDS solution; thick arrows with large heads are resultants (drift vectors)

Fig. 5.3 MDS with drift vectors for Morse code confusion data

The confusion probabilities are not symmetric. For example, the signal for i (di-di) is more frequently confused with a subsequent signal for s (di-di-di) than s is confused with a subsequent i (35% vs. 16%). But do these asymmetries exhibit a systematic pattern or are they just random? We answer this question using the `driftVectors()` function of the SMACOF package[2]:

```
data(morse2)   ## morse2 = 1 - confusion probabilities
fit.drift <- driftVectors(morse2, type="ordinal")
fit.drift
plot(fit.drift)
```

The solution is shown in Fig. 5.3. The configuration of points represents the symmetric part of the data quite well (Stress = 0.192). The resultant drift vectors form a vector field that indeed exhibits a systematic trend: All arrows point more or less into the same direction. Substantively, this means that long signals are more often confused with short ones than vice versa (see p. 70f. for more information on these data).

---

[2]Note that for converting a complete $n \times n$ matrix of similarities, **P**, into dissimilarities, you cannot use `sim2diss()`, because it does not work on the whole matrix. Use your own conversion. For example, run `diss <- max(P) - P`, and then use `diss` in `driftVectors`.

5.4   Modeling Individual Differences in MDS

A popular variant of MDS is the *dimensional weighting model*, often called the IND-SCAL model by the name of its original computer program (Carroll and Chang 1970). We explain the basic idea of this model using an experiment on color perception. Helm (1964) asked a sample of test persons to assess the similarity of ten chips with different colors (same brightness and same saturation). For each individual, similarity scores were obtained for each pair of colors. Some test persons were deuteranopic to some extent; i.e., they were not able to clearly distinguish green and purplish-red ("red-green blind").

Rather than first averaging the 16 data sets and then scaling the averaged data with standard MDS, we can use them directly in the dimensional weighting model. In this approach, we have to assume that there exists a *group space*, $\mathbf{X}$, that represents what all persons have in common. Moreover, each individual i has his/her individual space, $\mathbf{X}_i$. The model claims that the various individuals in the sample are not really that different. Rather, each *individual space* is a simple transform of the group space. That is, $\mathbf{X}_i = \mathbf{X}\mathbf{W}_i$, where $\mathbf{W}_i$ is a diagonal matrix with positive elements. Geometrically, this means that person i's individual space is generated by stretching or compressing the group space along its dimensions. INDSCAL fits this model by searching for both an $\mathbf{X}$ and for a set of weight matrices $\mathbf{W}_i$ such that the distances among the rows of the $\mathbf{X}_i$'s optimally correspond to the (admissibly transformed) dissimilarities of the persons (the dhat's). Expressed more formally, the distances are

$$d_{ijk}(\mathbf{X}) = \left(\sum_{a=1}^{m} w_{ak}(x_{ia} - x_{ja})^2 \right)^{1/2}, \qquad w_{ak} \geq 0, \qquad (5.5)$$

where the parameter $k = 1, ..., N$ stands for different individuals or cases.

For the Helm data, the group space (using SMACOF; see commands below) is computed as presented in the left panel of Fig. 5.4: It is the expected color circle, slightly squeezed in the vertical direction as the fitted circle (dashed line) shows. The middle panel contains the model's solution for the most deuteranopic person CD4: Here, the color circle is stretched along Dimension 1 or, which has the same effect, it is compressed along Dimension 2. This reflects that this person cannot discriminate well between green and the purplish-red colors. The right panel exhibits the solution for person N6a. This person, a color-normal person, stretches the group space somewhat along Dimension 2.

```
1  res.helm <- indscal(helm, type="interval")
2  res.helm  ## gives Stress-1 etc.
3  plot(res.helm)  ## plots the group space
4  names(res.helm)  ## shows elements of object res.helm
5  res.helm$cweights[[16]]  ## prints weight matrix for person 16
```

The weights for the 16 data sets are visualized in Fig. 5.5, often called the *subject space* of an INDSCAL solution. We here see that person CD4 stretches the group

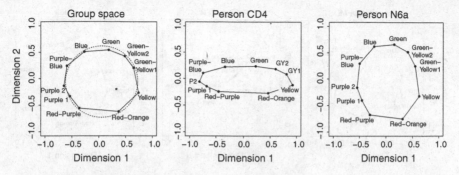

Fig. 5.4 Dimensional weighting MDS for Helm color data: group space (left panel); weighted group spaces of person CD4 who is red-green-deficient (middle); person N6a (right)

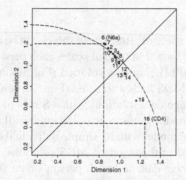

Fig. 5.5 Dimension weights of 16 individuals for group space shown in Fig. 5.4, left panel

space along Dimension 1 relative to Dimension 2 by a factor of roughly 3 (1.25 : 0.44). The weight ratio of person N6a is about 2:3. One must be careful, though, in interpreting these weights: They are only meaningful *relative to the group space*, and the group space is, unfortunately, *not unique*. If the group space is stretched or compressed along its dimensions, different weights are found for each person, while the overall fit of the MDS solution remains the same. What one can interpret as data-driven, therefore, is merely that person CD4 weights the vertical dimension less than person N6a, since this relation remains invariant under horizontal or vertical stretchings of the group space. That N6a weights Dimension 2 three times as much as CD4, or that he/she weights the dimensions in a certain weight ratio, is only true relative to the group space in Fig. 5.4. This also explains why the color-normal person N6a seems to put more weight on Dimension 2: The reason is that the group space also contains the data of the color-deficient persons which makes the configuration somewhat elliptical rather than circular as it would be true for color-normal persons only.

The overall Stress of the INDSCAL solution with its 2d group space for the ten colors and its sixteen 2×2 diagonal weight matrices is .123. The output object `res.helm` contains additional fit indexes such as Stress-per-Point measures. Most important is the fit of each person in this model. Here we find for person CD4 a Stress value of

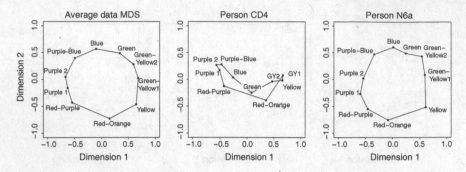

Fig. 5.6 Three separate standard interval MDS solutions for average color data, person's CD3 data, and person's N6a data, respectively; configurations of CD3 and N6a Procrustean-fitted to average data solution

.106 and for person N6a a value of .108. These values can be compared, for example, with the Stress values of standard MDS that scales each person's data separately. For the averaged data, interval MDS finds a solution (Fig. 5.6, left panel) with a Stress of .069. For person CD4, MDS finds a solution (Fig. 5.6, center panel; configuration Procrustean-fitted to average data solution) with a Stress of .074, and for N6a with .069. Thus, the INDSCAL model seems to be doing quite well and one could hope that the dimensional weighting model with its simple individual differences theory irons out error that is over-fitted in the standard MDS solutions. On the other hand, the results of scaling the average data and each person's data separately with standard MDS lead to essentially the same substantive insights.

If one drops the idea of common dimensions for all individuals,[3] a new model arises, the IDIOSCAL model (also called subjective metric model, elliptical distances model, or subjective transformations model). It admits more general person-specific transformations of the group space. Formally, in $\mathbf{XW}_i = \mathbf{X}_i$, the matrix $\mathbf{W}_i$ is *not* restricted to be diagonal, but can be any real-valued $m \times m$ matrix. Such a matrix can be interpreted in various ways. One interpretation is that person i first rotates the dimensions of the common space in his/her own way and then stretches/compresses the space along these dimensions.[4] Yet, such a transformation demolishes the major selling point of the INDSCAL model, namely its *unique* dimensions. Not only has an INDSCAL solution the *same* dimensions for *all* individuals, but *any* rotation of these dimensions generally leads to higher Stress. Users of INDSCAL—market researchers in particular—had always hoped that these dimensions were the "true" psychological dimensions underlying the observations.

---

[3]Computationally, this is done by requesting `constraint="idioscal"` in the `smacofIndDiff()` function or by simply using the `idioscal()` function.

[4]$\mathbf{W}_i$ can always be (uniquely) split by singular value decomposition into the product $\mathbf{UDV}'$, where $\mathbf{U}$ and $\mathbf{V}'$ are rotations/reflections, and $\mathbf{D}$ is a diagonal matrix of dimension weights. Hence, $\mathbf{XW}_i = \mathbf{XUDV}'$ means the group space is first rotated/reflected by $\mathbf{U}$, then weighted by $\mathbf{D}$, and then rotated once more.

In the example above, *meaningful* dimensions were indeed identified, but one should not expect that this will always be the case, simply because such dimensions may not exist. The user should also know that the fit of the INDSCAL model is not necessarily much worse if all dimension weights are set to the same value. Borg and Lingoes (1978) report an example where the dimension weights scatter substantially even though they explain very little additional variance over unit weights. In such a case, the unique orientation of the dimensions is not very strong either.

The idea of the dimension weighting model can also be realized in a more step-wise and bottom-up approach. This avoids some of the interpretation problems. To do this, one first scales each of the given N data matrices, one by one, by standard MDS. One then uses Procrustean transformations (see Sect. 7.6 on p. 84f. for details) to fit the N resulting configurations to each other by admissible transformations (rotations, reflections, size adjustments, and translations). The average of all the fitted configurations is then taken as the "common" configuration (*centroid configuration*), or, alternatively, one uses the MDS configuration based on the averaged data as the group space. Subsequently, one identifies the dimensions of the group space that, if weighted, optimally explain the individual MDS solutions. This *hierarchical* approach is used by the Procrustean-Individual-Differences-Scaling (PINDIS) model (Lingoes and Borg 1978). It also continues the bottom-up fitting process with IDIOSCAL and other more general models, all of them not very useful in practice. However, the hierarchical approach suggests checking how much better the fit of a more general model is compared to one with more restrictions. The user can ask such a question using the `smacofIndDiff()` function by first running the above script with `constraint="identity"` (see next section for more on that option), then with `constraint="indscal"`, and finally with `constraint="idioscal"`. The three resulting solutions have Stress values of .146, .123, and .121, respectively. So, for the Helm color data, individual dimension weighting leads to a noticeable Stress reduction, but admitting more general idiosyncratic transformations is hardly worth it.

5.5   Scaling Replicated Proximities

In most MDS applications, we are dealing with exactly one data value per distance. Modern MDS programs allow using not just one proximity (p_{ij}) for each distance d_{ij} but two or more ($p_{ij}^{(k)}$, $k = 1, 2, ...$). Consider Fig. 5.7, a stack of $n \times n$ complete proximity matrices. Often, the values in such a data cube are first averaged over all persons and then averaged once more over the two halves of the resulting complete matrix. The data in the rectangle experiment described on p. 19 were generated in this fashion. Alternatively, we could inform the MDS program that what we have is one complete data matrix for each of N persons and that we want the program to find a solution where each d_{ij} represents, as precisely as possible, up to $N \cdot (n^2 - n)$ proximities, where the "up to" means that missing data are possible. Only the main

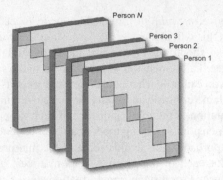

Fig. 5.7 Data cube consisting of complete proximity matrices for N persons

diagonals in each proximity matrix can *never* impact the MDS solution because $d_{ii} = 0$, for any i, is true in any distance geometry.

As an example, consider two sets of inter-correlations among work values collected in West and East Germany, respectively (see p. 84 for more on these data). These data can be loaded by calling data(EW_eng) in SMACOF: This activates a list of two correlation matrices, one for West Germany and the other for East Germany. If we interpret the entries in these correlation matrices as replications or as indicators of common German work value constructs, we could first average these matrices and then scale the averaged correlations. However, this reduces the number of data that determine the MDS solution in half, and more data for each distance should lead to a more data-driven, more robust solution. To use both matrices to generate one MDS solution, we can run this:

```
1  EW.diss <- list(east = sim2diss(EW_eng$east), west = sim2diss(EW_eng$west))
2  res <- smacofIndDiff(EW.diss, type="ordinal", constraint="identity")
3  res; summary(res)  ## gives Stress, coordinates, SPP values
4  plot(res, main="East+West combined")
```

5.6 Weighting Proximities in MDS

We saw in formula 3.3 that introducing weights into the MDS loss function is easily possible. It is always used if there are missing data, because then these weights are set to zero in case of an NA value. This makes the MDS algorithm ignore the distances that correspond to (missing) proximities. The distances can take on any value without affecting the Stress of the solution. However, for real data, one sometimes has additional information about the data such as their reliability. In that case, one may want to weight the more reliable data more in the Stress function. Another case is the size of the data themselves. Judgments on the similarity of pairs of objects are sometimes said to be the more difficult the more similar the objects are. The error that this uncertainty introduces can be expressed by weighting observed dissimilarities the heavier the greater they are. In other words, larger dissimilarities should determine the MDS solution more than smaller dissimilarities.

Computationally, weighting an MDS or an unfolding solution can be easily accomplished by adding a weight matrix of the size of the data matrix to the call of the MDS function or program. For example, assume we want to scale the inter-correlations in Table 2.2, **R**, and assume further that we have a table of reliabilities of these correlations, **W**. To run weighted MDS, we first have to convert the correlations into dissimilarities by `diss <- sim2diss(R)` and then call `result <- mds(diss, weightmat=W)`.

If you experiment with different weight matrices, you will find, though, that weights need considerable variance to affect the MDS configurations. One possibility is setting `W <- R^q` for some large or small `q`. For example, for `q=10` the large similarities (i.e., small dissimilarities) will be fitted much better than small similarities (i.e., large dissimilarities) so that only the small distances in the plot should be interpreted and the large distances be better ignored. For a very small `q`, e.g., `q=-10` the reverse is true. Hence, weighting can be useful in practice but it may require some experimentation. The Shepard diagram will show which dissimilarities are well fitted and which are not.

5.7   Summary

MDS is a family of different models. They differ in the way they map the proximities into distances, and in the distance functions they employ. The various regression functions preserve certain properties of the data such as the ranks of the data in ordinal MDS, the relative differences of any two data values in interval MDS, and the ratios of the data in ratio MDS. Typically, Euclidean distances are chosen as the targets in MDS. City-block distances or dominance metrics are also used in psychological modeling. Some MDS models allow using multiple proximities per distance. Asymmetric proximities can be handled by the drift vector model: It represents their symmetric part by the distances of an MDS configuration, and their skew-symmetric part by drift vectors attached to the points. A popular MDS model is INDSCAL which represents a set of N proximity matrices, one for each of N individuals, by one common MDS space and by N sets of individual weights for its dimensions.

References

Borg, I., & Lingoes, J. C. (1978). What weight should weights have in individual differences scaling? *Quality and Quantity, 12*, 223–237.

Carroll, J. D., & Chang, J. J. (1970). Analysis of individual differences in multidimensional scaling via an n-way generalization of 'Eckart-Young' decomposition. *Psychometrika, 35*, 283–320.

Helm, C. E. (1964). Multidimensional ratio scaling analysis of perceived color relations. *Journal of the Optical Society of America, 54*, 256–262.

Lingoes, J. C., & Borg, I. (1978). A direct approach to individual differences scaling using increasingly complex transformations. *Psychometrika*, *43*, 491–519.

Mair, P., Borg, I., & Rusch, T. (2016). Goodness-of-fit assessment in multidimensional scaling and unfolding. *Multivariate Behavioral Research*, *51*, 772–789.

Rothkopf, E. Z. (1957). A measure of stimulus similarity and errors in some paired-associate learning. *Journal of Experimental Psychology*, *53*, 94–101.

Torgerson, W. S. (1952). Multidimensional scaling: I. Theory and method. *Psychometrika*, *17*, 401–419.

Weeks, D. G., & Bentler, P. M. (1979). A comparison of linear and monotone multidimensional scaling models. *Psychological Bulletin*, *86*, 349–354.

Chapter 6
Confirmatory MDS

Abstract Different forms of confirmatory MDS are introduced, from weak forms
with external starting configurations to enforcing theoretical constraints onto the
MDS point coordinates or onto certain regions of the MDS space.

Keywords Confirmatory MDS · External scales · Dimensional constraints
Shearing · Axial partition · Penalty function

In the MDS models discussed so far, the computer was free to move the points
to any positions in space that would minimize the configuration's Stress. This is
exploratory MDS. If one has clear hypotheses about the MDS configuration, one
may be less interested in blindly minimizing Stress, but rather in finding an optimal
theory-consistent MDS solution. This leads to *confirmatory* MDS.

6.1 Weak Confirmatory MDS

The least one can do when testing structural theories using MDS is running the MDS
with an external initial configuration derived from theory rather than leaving it to
the program to choose its own start. This can help finding good solutions in the
vicinity of what is expected. One can also fit the MDS solutions thus obtained to
theory-based *target* configurations. For example, in case of the rectangle study from
Sect. 2.3, the design configuration of Fig. 2.4, appropriately stretched or compressed
along its dimensions, can serve both as an initial configuration and also as a target
in subsequent Procrustean transformations of the MDS configuration (see Sect. 7.6).

An external initial configuration can also help to make a set of different MDS
solutions more similar. Consider a study by Dichtl et al. (1980). These authors analyzed consumer perceptions of various automobiles collected year after year over
a period of five years. They first computed the MDS solution of the averaged data
and then used this configuration as the initial configuration when scaling each of the

five yearly data sets. This makes it more likely that the various solutions are more similar, because the MDS algorithm always begins its optimization process with the same configuration.

6.2   External Side Constraints on the Dimensions

A *strict* confirmatory MDS approach *enforces* a solution that satisfies the external constraints while minimizing Stress. The simplest such model is to impose certain restrictions onto dimensions that span the MDS space.

As an application example, we use the rectangle study from Sect. 2.3. Exploratory MDS of these data leads to a solution that closely approximates a psychologically reasonable transformation of the design grid (Fig. 2.5). We now employ confirmatory MDS to enforce such a grid *perfectly* onto the solution and then check whether this leads to Stress values that are still acceptably low. This can be realized by the smacofConstraint() function. It allows the user to request that an $n \times m$ MDS solution $\mathbf{X}$ is generated by optimally scaling the column vectors of an external $n \times m$ matrix $\mathbf{Y}$. For $\mathbf{Y}$, we here take the coordinates of the points in the design grid, i.e., their width and height measurements (see Fig. 2.4 or simply activate these data by data(rect_constr)). The columns of $\mathbf{Y}$ are called *external scales*, and after *optimal re-scaling*, they become the *internal scales*, the columns of $\mathbf{X}$.

Re-scaling can mean different things:

- In the simplest case, it means dimensional weighting. That is, the data are approximated, as much as possible, by the distances computed on a configuration whose dimensions are the optimally weighted columns of $\mathbf{Y}$. Expressed formally $\mathbf{X} = \mathbf{YC}$, with $\mathbf{C}$ a diagonal matrix that minimizes the Stress of $\mathbf{X}$.
- If we drop the constraint that $\mathbf{C}$ is diagonal, then $\mathbf{C}$ becomes a *composite* transformation. It can be understood as a rotation/reflection followed by dimensional weighting and then rotated/reflected once more. Thus, expressed geometrically, the dimensional weighting can be done along a *rotated* set of dimensions.
- A third case is allowing for optimal monotone transformations of $\mathbf{Y}$'s columns or of the columns of a rotated $\mathbf{Y}$.

For the rectangle data, the third model is theoretically most convincing. We test it by first running exploratory MDS and then plotting this solution with its points connected as a grid. Then, we use this solution as the initial configuration in confirmatory MDS,[1] enforcing an ordinal rescaling of the unrotated design dimensions. Finally, we also allow for a rotation of the design configuration.

---

[1]If no external initial configuration is provided, the program will use a random start. In most applications, this will not lead to low Stress nor to a meaningful solution.

```
1  ## MDS with theory-based initial configuration
2  fit.expl <- mds(rectangles, type = "ordinal", init = rect_constr)
3  ## MDS enforcing an ordinally re-scaled design grid
4  fit.cfdiag <- smacofConstraint(rectangles, constraint = "diagonal",
5                  type = "ordinal", ties = "secondary",
6                  init = fit.expl$conf, external = rect_constr,
7                  constraint.type = "ordinal")
8  ## Confirmatory MDS, also permitting a rotation of the design grid
9  fit.cflin  <- smacofConstraint(rectangles, constraint = "linear",
10                  type = "ordinal", ties = "secondary",
11                  init = fit.expl$conf, external = rect_constr,
12                  constraint.type = "ordinal")
```

Figure 6.1 shows the resulting configurations. The exploratory MDS solution (left panel) is already nearly theory-compatible except for some small dents of the grid. Its Stress is 0.089. The first confirmatory solution (middle panel) is theory-wise perfect, with a Stress of 0.115. Hence, the dents of the grid in the exploratory MDS solution do not explain the data "much" better. Rather, it seems that they essentially represent some of the data noise. So, one may decide not to reject the hypothesis that the observed judgments for the rectangles' similarity are generated by a composition rule that behaves just like the distance formula operating on the rectangles' design dimensions.

If we drop the diagonality constraint on **C**, we get the *sheared* grid in the right panel of Fig. 6.1. Its Stress is 0.103, slightly better than without the rotation. It suggests that not the original dimensions were rescaled but a slightly rotated (but theoretically obscure) dimension system. This causes the shearing of the grid. (In practice, such shearings can become extreme in this model which make the solutions difficult to interpret.)

If we set `constraint.type="interval"`, the transformations on the design grid are limited to stretchings of the external scales, i.e., to simple dimensional weightings (plus possible shearings). Under this condition, the successively smaller compressions of the grid along its dimensions generated by `constraint.type="ordinal"`

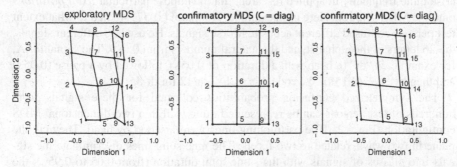

Fig. 6.1 Exploratory (left) MDS of rectangle data of Sect. 2.3; and confirmatory MDS of the same data with stretchings of the given dimensions (center panel) and with stretchings of rotated dimensions (right panel)

cannot occur anymore in the MDS solution. This would be undesirable here, because the Weber–Fechner law of perception is predicting such logarithmic shrinkage effects.

Returning to the model equation $\mathbf{X} = \mathbf{YC}$, we note that the matrix $\mathbf{C}$ represents a *linear transformation* of the configuration $\mathbf{Y}$. Any linear transformation can be decomposed into rotations and dimensional weightings of $\mathbf{Y}$. Algebraically, that means that $\mathbf{C}$ can be split by singular value decomposition into the product $\mathbf{PMQ}$, where $\mathbf{P}$ and $\mathbf{Q}$ represent rotations and $\mathbf{M}$ is a diagonal matrix of dimension weights. Thus, $\mathbf{C}$ first rotates the configuration $\mathbf{Y}$ in some way and then stretches and/or compresses this *rotated* configuration along its dimensions and finally rotates the result once more. If $\mathbf{C}$ is a diagonal matrix, then the column vectors of $\mathbf{Y}$ are weighted directly. If $\mathbf{C}$ is not diagonal, then $\mathbf{Y}$ is first rotated and then dimensionally weighted, and this is what causes the shearing.

A different approach to impose external constraints onto the MDS solution is to focus on the distances of the MDS configuration, not on its coordinates. If, for example, one requests for the rectangle data that $d(1, 6) = d(2, 5)$, $d(6, 11) = d(7, 10)$, and $d(11, 16) = d(12, 15)$ must hold in the MDS solution, shearings of the point grid are avoided. To guarantee that a grid is generated in the first place, one can additionally enforce that some of the horizontal grid distances be equally long, e.g., that $d(1, 5) = d(2, 6) = d(3, 7) = d(4, 8)$, $d(5, 9) = d(6, 10) = d(7, 11) = d(8, 12)$, and $d(9, 13) = d(10, 14) = d(11, 15) = d(12, 16)$. Restrictions like these can be imposed on the MDS configuration by the program CMDA (Borg and Lingoes 1980). CMDA is, unfortunately, an old Fortran program that is not easily accessible and difficult to use because it is not always easy to derive what a given theory implies for the distances among the points in MDS space.

6.3   Regional Axial Restrictions

One can use the methods discussed above to solve confirmatory MDS problems that arise quite frequently in applied research, that is, impose particular *axial partitions* onto the MDS solution. Here is an example. Rothkopf (1957) studied to what extent test persons confused different acoustic Morse signals. He used 36 different signals, the 26 letters of the alphabet, and the natural numbers from 0 to 9. The signal for A, for example, is "di" (a beep with a duration of 0.05 s), followed by a pause (0.05 s) and then by "da" (0.15 s). We code this as 1–2 or 12 for di-da.

The symmetrized confusion probabilities collected for these signals from hundreds of test persons can be represented quite well in a two-dimensional MDS configuration (Fig. 6.2). The partitioning lines were inserted by hand. They cut the plane in two ways, related to two facets: The nine solid lines discriminate the signals into classes of signals with the same total duration (from 0.05 to 0.95 s); the five dashed lines separate the signals on the basis of their composition (e.g., signals containing only long beeps are all on the right-hand side). The pattern of these partitioning lines is not very simple, though, but partially rather curvy and hard to

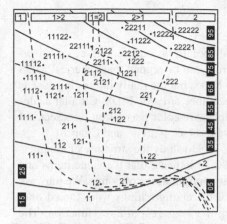

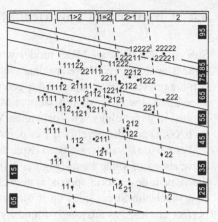

Fig. 6.2 Exploratory MDS representation for 36 Morse signals; lines correspond to two typologies for the signals

Fig. 6.3 Confirmatory MDS solution with two perfect axial partitioning lines

describe. Particularly, the dashed lines are so twisted that the pattern of the emerging regions does not exhibit a simple law of formation. Rather, the partitioning seems over-fitted. The substantive researcher, therefore, would probably not bet that it can be completely replicated with new data.

We now want to straighten the two sets of partitioning lines. For that purpose, we again use the $\mathbf{X} = \mathbf{YC}$ restriction. To generate the internal scales in $\mathbf{X}$, we make use of two of the signal codes' properties, duration and type, as shown in Fig. 6.2 by the vertical black boxes (duration) and the boxes on top labeled as "1", "1 > 2", "1 = 2", "2 < 1", and "2" (type). Each Morse code is thus coded in terms of its duration into one of ten categories and in terms of type into one of five categories. This defines the external variables, $\mathbf{Y}$. They can be viewed by typing data(morsescales); morsescales in SMACOF.

With these constraints in an ordinal MDS, with ordinal external scales, and with the primary approach to ties, we find the solution in Fig. 6.3. This simple-to-interpret MDS solution has almost the same overall Stress as the exploratory MDS solution in Fig. 6.2 (0.21 vs. 0.18). Upon closer investigation one notes, however, that the confirmatory solution moved only very few points by more than a small amount. Particularly, point 1 (at the bottom, to the right) was moved a lot so that the substantive researcher may want to study this signal (and its relationship to other stimuli such as signal 2) more closely. Overall, though, the simpler and, probably, also more replicable solution in Fig. 6.3 appears to be the better springboard for further research.

6.4   Circular and Spherical MDS

Spherical MDS is an MDS model where all points lie on the surface of an m-dimensional sphere. There are data sets where it can be argued that spherical MDS is more relevant than the usual flat-geometry MDS, but the really interesting case is $m = 2$, i.e., the case where spherical MDS becomes *circular* MDS. Circular scales abound in psychology. Two prominent examples are color perception (see Sect. 5.4 on p. 60ff.) and the psychology of personal values (see p. 21ff., and Chap. 8).

For personal values, we used exploratory MDS to study the structure of the inter-correlations of value items. Figures 2.10 and 2.13 indicate that the value items and the value indexes form approximately circular configurations of points. We may ask how much the Stress goes up if the points of the configurations were forced onto perfect circles. An answer is found by using the smacofSphere() function: The Stress of the exploratory solution is 0.051; it goes up to 0.085 in the perfect-circle solution.

Enforcing a perfect circle for these data does, however, not really lead to new insights, since the exploratory configuration is already roughly circular. Moreover, a perfect circle is not needed for indexes that are based on real and therefore error-affected data. To see more dramatic or unexpected effects, let us therefore request a circular MDS configuration for the similarity of countries data represented in Fig. 2.2. Since there is no substantive reason to enforce a circle, we should expect that this constraint entails a substantial increment in Stress.

When running this type of analysis with smacofSphere(), we have a choice of two algorithms: The primal algorithm enforces a strict circle from the beginning, and the dual algorithm uses a penalty function that pushes the MDS solution in the direction of a perfect circle. The default penalty weight is 100, and when setting it to 22, say, the force that pulls the solution toward a perfect circle is mitigated. Let us try both specifications as follows:

```
 1  diss <- sim2diss(wish, method=max(wish))
 2  res1 <- smacofSphere(diss, type="ordinal")
 3  res2 <- smacofSphere(diss, type="ordinal", algorithm="dual", penalty=22)
 4  res3 <- mds(diss)
 5  res1$stress; res2$stress; res3$stress ## gives Stress values of each solution
 6  op <- par(mfrow = c(1,3))
 7  plot(res1, main="Circular MDS (primal)")
 8  plot(res2, main="Circular MDS 2 (dual)")
 9  plot(res3, main="Exploratory MDS")
10  par(op)
```

The three results are shown in Fig. 6.4. As expected, the solution generated by the default algorithm (algorithm="primal") has all country points on a perfect circle, while the solution computed by the dual algorithm and using penality=22 only comes close to a perfect circle. When setting the penalty weight to 100 (i.e., the default value), then the circle is perfect too. So, we see that choosing smaller penalty weights is a way to avoid that the algorithm is pushing too hard toward a perfect circle.

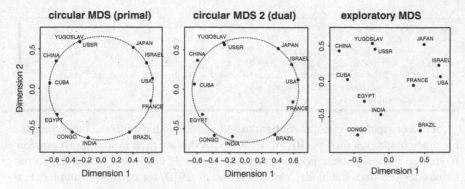

Fig. 6.4 Circular MDS using the primal and the dual algorithm, resp., and exploratory MDS (right panel) of Wish country similarity data

The Stress values for the solutions in Fig. 6.4 are 0.271, 0.266, and 0.225, respectively. The increment in Stress is not much higher than it is in case of the personal values example discussed above, even though now there are 12 points and not just 10 points. However, one should take into account that the Stress for the Wish data is quite high even without circular side constraints. Nevertheless, when studying the three plots more closely, one can indeed see that the exploratory MDS solution is not that far from being circular: Only France needs to be pulled somewhat to the outside and Congo more toward the center of the plot. Whether a circular configuration for the countries is substantively meaningful is, of course, another question.

When testing theories about real data, forcing the points onto a perfect circle in MDS space may seem exaggerated formalism. An approximate circle would be sufficient, but it is much harder to formulate this idea as a clear scaling target. Moreover, a perfect circle is, by itself, rarely ever a meaningful structural theory. It only becomes interesting if it is supplemented with additional notions such as a particular order of the points on the circle. In case of the data on personal values (see p. 25), the Theory on Universals in Values (Schwartz 1992) predicts such an order. The theory also claims that the point order is structured into four subsets of opposite higher-order personal values. This would split the circle into four arcs that lie in four different quadrants. If you have inter-correlations as data, circular scaling solutions with various additional constraints can be generated using the R package CIRCE (Grassi et al. 2010). This program implements the Guttman–Browne circumplex model for inter-correlations (Browne 1992). It assumes that an observed correlation r_{ij} corresponds to an angle between the vectors pointing to the points i and j on a unit circle. The method does not accept order constraints, but they can be approximated to some extent by restricting the points to lie in certain sectors of the circle. For example, with the personal values grouped into four higher-order values, and the PVQ40 data aggregated into ten indices as in the first 11 lines of the R script on p. 23, the R commands are:

```
1  require(CircE); R <- cor(PVQ40agg)
2  ## CircE commands (with lots of default agruments):
3  lower1 <- c(0,0,0,270,270,180,180,180,90,90) ## lower bounds for point angles
4  upper1 <- c(90,90,90,360,360,270,270,270,180,180) ## upper bounds
5  res <- CircE.BFGS(R, v.names=colnames(R), m=1, N=10, upper=upper1, lower=
        lower1, equal.com=FALSE, equal.ang=FALSE)
6  CircE.Plot(res, ef=0.1)
```

CircE computes a circular configuration together with extensive output, including many fit indexes such as GIF, AGIF, RMSEA that are used in structural equation modeling. They test the hypothesis that the observed correlations match the correlations derived from the model. See (Grassi et al. 2010) for detailed examples. For the above PVQ40 data, the fit is highly significant, and the results are quite similar to what is shown in Fig. 2.13.

6.5 Challenges of Confirmatory MDS

The challenges of confirmatory MDS for the user are, most of all, how to formulate theoretical expectations so that they can be expressed in, say, a penalty function, a pseudo-data matrix, or a system of equations that can be solved by an existing confirmatory MDS program. Confirmatory MDS, therefore, is often much harder than exploratory MDS, because it requires the user to not only develop explicit theories but also translating them into a proper computational language. So far, the MDS programs accessible to the general user can handle only relatively simple confirmatory analyses. Dimensional restrictions are easy to test, while confirmatory MDS analyses with regional restrictions are typically difficult to set up and solve. Computer programs that allow all forms of restrictions (combined, in addition, with particular MDS models, certain missing data patterns, or distances other than Euclidean distances) do not exist yet. Rather, in such cases, a suitable MDS algorithm must be programmed ad hoc.

If the users succeed generating a confirmatory MDS solution, a number of additional challenges await them. They have to evaluate not only the absolute Stress values, but also the Stress increment resulting from adding the particular external constraints to the MDS analysis. Typically, such evaluations amount to deciding whether the Stress increment is substantial or not, given the number of points, the dimensionality of the MDS space, the MDS model, the distance function, and the quality of the data (error level). These and further criteria are summarized by Lingoes and Borg (1983) in a quasi-statistical decision procedure.

An important additional criterion is the strength of the external constraints. These constraints may be easy to satisfy for a given number of points in a given dimensionality, but they may also be quite demanding. An approach for evaluating this issue is described in Borg et al. (2011). They use data from a survey where a sample of employees assessed 54 organizational culture themes (e.g., "being competitive," "working long hours," and "being careful") in terms of how important they are for them personally. The correlations of these importance ratings are represented in a theory-compatible MDS solution, where the 54 points are forced into the quadrants of a 2d coordinate system on the basis of a priori codings of the items in terms of the TUV theory. The strength of the external constraints is assessed by studying the Stress values that result from running 1,000 different confirmatory MDS analyses, each one using a random permutation of these TUV codings. It is found that the theory-based assignment of codes to the 54 items does indeed lead to a Stress value that is smaller than any of the Stress values that are found if random permutations of the codings are enforced onto the MDS solution. Hence, the codings are *not trivial* in the sense that random assignments of the codings would lead to equally good MDS solutions when enforced onto the configuration.

6.6 Summary

MDS is mostly used in an exploratory way, where the MDS configuration is chosen so that the Stress is minimal. Confirmatory MDS enforces additional structure onto the MDS space, or it at least tries to push the solution toward a theoretically expected structure. Confirmatory MDS configurations may be very different from exploratory MDS solutions. Often, their Stress is higher, but sometimes it is not. Without running confirmatory MDS, one would not know. A weak way to push an MDS solution toward a theoretical structure is using a theory-derived initial configuration. Harder confirmatory requirements need special MDS programs such as PROXSCAL or `smacofConstraint`. With such programs, one can enforce certain dimensional requirements and strict axial partitionings. Circular configurations require spherical MDS programs such as `smacofSphere()` or `CircE`.

References

Borg, I., Groenen, P. J. F., Jehn, K. A., Bilsky, W., & Schwartz, S. H. (2011). Embedding the organizational culture profile into Schwartz's theory of universals in values. *Journal of Personnel Psychology*, *10*, 1–12.

Borg, I., & Lingoes, J. C. (1980). A model and algorithm for multidimensional scaling with external constraints on the distances. *Psychometrika*, *45*, 25–38.

Browne, M. W. (1992). Circumplex models for correlation matrices. *Psychometrika*, *57*, 469–497.

Dichtl, E., Bauer, H. H., & Schobert, R. (1980). Die Dynamisierung mehrdimensionaler Marktmodelle am Beispiel des deutschen Automobilmarkts. *Marketing*, *3*, 163–177.

Grassi, M., Luccio, R., & Di Blas, L. (2010). CircE: An R implementation of Browne's circular stochastic process model. *Behavior Research Methods*, *42*, 55–73.

Lingoes, J. C., & Borg, I. (1983). A quasi-statistical model for choosing between alternative configurations derived from ordinally constrained data. *British Journal of Mathematical and Statistical Psychology*, *36*, 36–53.

Rothkopf, E. Z. (1957). A measure of stimulus similarity and errors in some paired-associate learning. *Journal of Experimental Psychology*, *53*, 94–101.
Schwartz, S. H. (1992). Universals in the content and structure of values: Theoretical advances and empirical tests in 20 countries. *Advances in Experimental Social Psychology*, *25*, 1–65.

Chapter 7
Typical Mistakes in MDS

Abstract Various mistakes that users tend to make when using MDS are discussed, from using MDS for the wrong type of data, using MDS programs with suboptimal specifications, to misinterpreting MDS solutions.

Keywords Global optimum · Local optimum · Termination criterion
Initial configuration · Degenerate solution · Dimensional interpretation
Regional interpretation · Procrustean transformation

7.1 Assigning the Wrong Polarity to Proximities

A frequent beginner's mistake is scaling proximities with the wrong polarity. If the data are similarities, but MDS treats them as dissimilarities (or vice versa), it will generate a misleading solution with very high Stress. The MDS program cannot know how to interpret the data and, therefore, works with its default interpretation of the data. This usually means that the data are taken as dissimilarities. Yet, correlations, for example, are similarities, because greater correlation coefficients indicate higher similarity and, therefore, they should be represented by relatively small distances. If the user incorrectly specifies the data's polarity, then MDS cannot generate meaningful solutions.

7.2 Using Too Few Iterations

Many MDS programs have suboptimal default specifications. In particular, they typically terminate the iterations of their optimization algorithms before the process has actually converged at a local minimum. This premature termination is caused by setting the termination criteria too defensively. Many programs set the maximum number of iterations to 100 or less, a specification that dates back to the times when computing was slow and expensive. For example, the GUI box of SYSTAT in Fig. 1.5 shows that, per default, this MDS program allows at most 50 iterations. The iterations are also stopped if the Stress does not go down by more than 0.005 per iteration. However, one can show that very small Stress reductions do not always mean that all points remain essentially fixed in further iterations. We therefore recommend to always *clearly* change these default values to allow the program to work longer. Instead of a maximum of 50 one can easily require 1,000 or more iterations. The convergence criterion, in turn, could be set to 0.000001 or smaller, i.e., to a very small value indeed.

7.3   Using the Wrong Initial Configuration

All MDS programs automatically generate their own initial configuration if the user does not provide an external starting configuration. It is a common fallacy to assume that internally generated starting configurations will always lead to optimal MDS solutions. For example, we have found in many tests that the default starting configuration used in PROXSCAL (called "SIMPLEX") is often not optimal. We recommend using the option INITIAL=TORGERSON instead. Yet, *no* starting configuration—rational or user-provided—always guarantees the best-possible final solution, and so the user should test some sensible alternatives before accepting a particular MDS solution all too early as the final solution.

Random starting configurations can also be useful in MDS. Indeed, *many* random configurations can easily be used without much effort. For example, for the solution in Fig. 1.4 we used PROXSCAL with the option RANDOM=1000; i.e., we asked the program to repeat the scaling with 1,000 different random starting configurations and then report the solution with the lowest Stress value. That only took seconds with this small data set.

The same method can also be used with mds() in SMACOF. However, mds() generates only 1 random configuration when setting the argument init="random" in mds(). Thus, we have to program a loop to find the best solution or use the function random.multistart() below (which here calls an ordinal MDS and 500 random starts):

```
1  diss <- sim2diss(wish, method=7)
2  set.seed(123)
3  random.multistart <- function(diss, type="ordinal", nrep=100) { s1 <- 1
4    for (i in 1:nrep) { out <- mds(diss, type=type, init="random")
5    if (out$stress < s1) { object <- out; s1 <- out$stress }}
6  return(object) }
7  result <- random.multistart(diss, type="ordinal", nrep=500)
8  result
```

Running the above commands leads to a result$stress of .185 for the country similarity data from Sect. 2.2. Repeating this analysis with different seeds leads to the same minimum Stress value in each case. So, .185 seems to be the best-possible Stress for ordinal MDS of these data.

Sometimes there exist several *different* solutions that all have *almost* the same small Stress value. In that case, the user can pick the solution that is most convincing in terms of interpretation. The problem is that all MDS computer programs only report the best solution they found, where "best" obviously only says that it has the smallest Stress. No program can consider a configuration's meaning as an additional criterion. To help finding possible solutions that have both an acceptable Stress but differ in their substantive meaningfulness, Borg and Mair (2017) suggest a strategy where all MDS solutions that result from many different initial configurations are stored and then compared with respect to their structural similarity. This strategy is implemented in the icExplore() function. It generates a large set of MDS solutions using random initial configurations, matches them all by Procrustean fittings, computes the inter-correlations of their point coordinates, and finally runs an (interval) MDS of these inter-correlations.

```
diss <- sim2diss(wish, method=7)
set.seed(3)
solutions <- icExplore(diss, type="ordinal", nrep=75)
solutions
plot(solutions)
```

The result of this analysis for the country similarity data using 75 random initial configurations is shown in Fig. 7.1. The numbers in the plot represent the MDS configurations, and the size of the numbers corresponds to the Stress of the solution (solution #64, thus, has a poor fit to the data). The distances among the points represent the similarities of the configurations. The plot thus shows that there are many different local minima solutions when random initial configurations are used. Many of these solutions have a poor fit, but there are two clusters of highly similar configurations on the right-hand side that all have relatively low Stress. The user can take a look at, say, #9 (in the upper cluster on the right-hand side of Fig. 7.1) and #25 (in the cluster underneath) to see how they differ and which one is better interpretable (see discussion in Sect. 7.8). One can plot #9, say, by simply calling plot(solutions[[9]]). The Stress is printed by solutions[[9]].

The user can also follow another strategy. Compute a Stress-optimal MDS solution first, study its interpretability, and then possibly move some points "by hand" to theoretically more pleasing positions. These hand movements can be translated into changes of the coordinates of these points. The modified coordinate matrix can subsequently be used as the initial configuration in Stress0(). This function computes the Stress of the modified solution (without any iterations). Alternatively, one may set niter=1000, for example, and hope that the program will find an optimal solution with an acceptably small Stress that lies in the vicinity of the modified configuration.

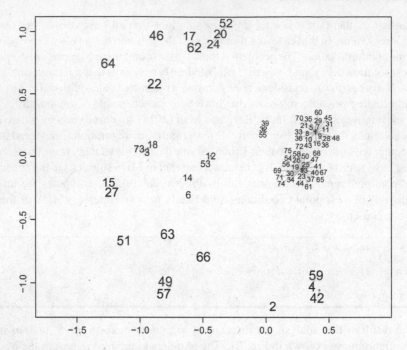

Fig. 7.1 Similarity structure of MDS solutions based on 75 random initial configurations for country similarity data; number represents solution; size of number represents Stress of solution

Finally, a theory-generated initial configuration (if it can be derived) is always a choice that should at least be tested. Consider, for example, the data on the similarity of rectangles and the data on personal values discussed in Chap. 2. In both cases, there were clear hypotheses about the expected MDS structure of the data. These predictions can easily be translated into coordinate matrices that then serve to define initial configurations. For example, for the rectangle data, one can simply read off the coordinates from Fig. 2.4 or call data(rect_constr); S <- rect_constr and then tell the MDS program to use **S** as an initial configuration.

There is usually no need to formulate the initial configuration as precisely as in case of matrix **S** above, nor does the theory always allow such precise predictions. This is certainly true for the personal values data, where the theory predicts a circle with points ordered as PO - AC - HE - ST - SD - UN - BE - TR - CO - SE - PO. No prediction can be derived for the distances among the points on the circle and so one could spread them out evenly, for example. It suffices to plot this configuration on a piece of paper, co-ordinatize its points by a simple grid, and then coarsely read off these coordinates to generate a matrix like **S** above. Of course, one could also do this on the computer screen, then plot the coordinate matrix to visually check it, and possibly adjust the point coordinates repeatedly until the configuration seems right.

7.4 Doing Nothing to Avoid Suboptimal Local Minima

MDS always tries to find the local minimum solution with the smallest possible Stress, i.e., the *global minimum*. MDS users can do their share to help find this global minimum by keeping an eye on the following issues:

- A good initial configuration is the best way to avoid suboptimal local minima. If you have a theory, then a user-defined configuration is what you should always use. If you do not have a theory, you must leave it to the MDS program to define its own starting configuration. In that case, we recommend using the solution of classical MDS (also known as the *Torgerson solution*) as a start which is indeed the default initial configuration of mds() in the SMACOF package.
- Another precaution against suboptimal local minima is using multiple random starts. As modern MDS programs are extremely fast, one can easily require the program to repeat the scaling with a very large number of different random starts (e.g., with 1,000 or more).
- City-block distances increase the risk to end up in suboptimal local minima. General MDS programs are particularly sensitive in this regard. There exist MDS programs that are optimized for city-block distances, but they are hard to obtain and typically require expert support for using them.
- The greater the dimensionality of the MDS space, the smaller the risk for suboptimal local minima. The main problem in low-dimensional spaces (1d, in particular) is that swapping points in space by iteratively repeating small movements is difficult, because such movements may first increase the Stress before it goes down. Hence, even if you want, say, a two-dimensional MDS solution, using the first two principal components of a three-dimensional MDS solution may serve as a good initial configuration.
- Suboptimal local minima are particularly likely in case of one-dimensional MDS. Standard programs almost never find the global minimum. If you must do one-dimensional MDS, you should provide an external starting configuration computed with 2d MDS (see above), or use an MDS program for the 1d case. Special 1d MDS programs are based on permutation algorithms which are computationally demanding. An example is uniscale() in the SMACOF package: It finds the permutation of the points with the smallest Stress, but always assumes that the data are on a ratio scale. Yet, one may use its solution as an initial configuration in ordinal and interval MDS.

7.5 Not Recognizing Degenerate Solutions

Of all MDS models, ordinal MDS is the model that has been used most often. It allows any rescaling of the data that preserves their order, but it nevertheless produces stable metric solutions. However, ordinal MDS can run into a special problem that the user should keep an eye on; i.e., it can lead to *degenerate* solutions. Consider the following example. Table 7.1 exhibits the inter-correlations of eight test items of

Table 7.1 Correlations (lower half) of some test items of the KIPT and their ranks (upper half).

	NP	LVP	SVP	CCP	NR	SLP	CCR	ILR
Nonsense word production (NP)	–	9	4	1	6	19	10	12
Long vowel production (LVP)	.78	–	1	7	5	21	20	22
Short vowel production (SVP)	.87	.94	–	3	2	17	16	23
Consonant cluster production (CCP)	.94	.83	.90	–	7	14	11	16
Nonsense word recognition (NR)	.84	.85	.91	.83	–	17	15	18
Single letter production (SLP)	.53	.47	.56	.60	.56	–	13	16
Consonant cluster recognition(CCR)	.72	.48	.57	.69	.59	.62	–	8
Initial letter recognition (ILR)	.66	.45	.44	.57	.55	.57	.82	–

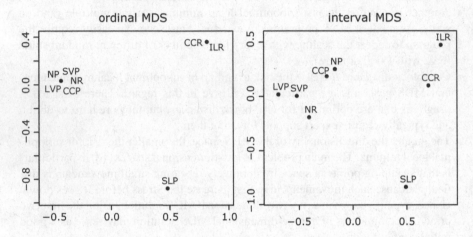

Fig. 7.2 Ordinal and interval MDS representations for data of Table 7.1

the Kennedy Institute Phonics Test (KIPT), a test for reading skills (Guthrie 1973). If we scale these data by ordinal MDS using mds() (see commands below[1]), we obtain the configuration in Fig. 7.2 (left panel). Its Stress value is zero, so this MDS solution is formally perfect. Yet, the Shepard diagram of this solution (see left panel of Fig. 7.3) reveals a peculiar relation of data and distances: Although the data scatter evenly over the interval from .44 to .94, they are not represented by distances with a similar distribution, but rather by two clearly distinct classes of distances so that the regression line makes just one big step.

```
1  diss <- sim2diss(KIPT)
2  fit1 <- mds(diss, type="ordinal", eps=1e-11)
3  fit2 <- mds(diss, type="interval")
4  fit3 <- mds(diss, type="ratio")
```

---

[1]Note that we set the argument eps to an extra-small value here to make the program iterate on and on until it reaches such an exotically small raw Stress value if it can be reached in itmax=3333 iterations. Without this argument, mds() will use the default value eps=1e-06 which causes it to stop earlier.

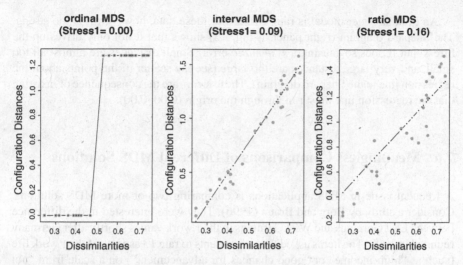

Fig. 7.3 Shepard diagrams for ordinal MDS, interval MDS, and ratio MDS of the correlations of Table 7.1 (converted into dissimilarities)

The MDS configuration shows three clusters that form an equilateral triangle. This configuration represents all large correlations ($r \geq .78$) by distances close to zero and all smaller correlations ($r < .72$) by the same large distance. This solution correctly displays a few data relations, but loses whatever else there is in the data. The perfect Stress value is, therefore, deceptive. The large and the small distances, respectively, *can be reordered arbitrarily* as long as all similarities within the blocks marked in Table 7.1 remain greater than all between-block similarities. Any such reordering will have no effect on the Stress value.

The reason for such a degenerate solution is that the data have a peculiar structure. They form three subgroups, with high within- and low between-correlations. With ordinal MDS, such data can always be scaled with zero Stress. Of course, the data here are particularly selected to demonstrate degeneracy. In practice, one should rarely find such cases, but the problem becomes more likely if the number of variables is small ($n \leq 8$).

If the Shepard diagram suggests that the MDS solution is degenerate, then the natural next step for the user is testing a *stronger* MDS model and comparing the solutions. Using interval MDS with the above data yields the solution in the right panel of Fig. 7.2. It too shows the three clusters of test items, but it does not collapse them. Its Shepard diagram (see the middle panel of Fig. 7.3) makes clear that the interval solution preserves a *linear* relationship of the data in Table 7.1 to the distances in Fig. 7.2.[2]

---

[2]Note that if you plot the correlations of Table 7.1 rather than the dissimilarities on the Y-axis of the Shepard diagram of the interval MDS—using plot(aus1, plot.type="Shepard", shepard.x=kipt)—the regression line is slightly curved. This is so because transforming the correlations into dissimilarities via $\delta_{ij} = \sqrt{1 - r_{ij}}$—which is what

An even stronger model is ratio MDS. For these data, however, it is too strong. The Shepard diagram (right panel of Fig. 7.3) shows that it not only drives up the Stress, but it does so causing a *systematic* error: Small distances are almost all too small, and very large distances are too large (see the scatter of the points about the regression line in the Shepard diagram). These errors are the consequence of insisting that the regression line must run through the origin (0.00, 0.00).

7.6 Meaningless Comparisons of Different MDS Solutions

A frequent issue in MDS applications is comparing two or more MDS solutions. Consider a study by Borg and Braun (1996). They were interested in the difference between East Germans and West Germans in their work values shortly after Germany reunited in 1990. The items asked the respondents to rate 13 aspects of their work life (such as "high income" or "good chances for advancement") on a scale from "not important" to "very important" to them personally. Scaling the inter-correlations of the two samples leads to two-dimensional MDS solutions, but even though they have just 13 points each, they are difficult to compare, because one must ignore *meaningless* differences that are due to different orientations of the plots. It is like comparing two maps of different size, and one is upside down, for example. When comparing MDS plots, one can eliminate such meaningless differences optimally by *Procrustean transformations*. If configuration **X** is taken as the target, the other configuration **Y** is rotated, reflected, translated, and adjusted in its size to optimally match **X**. All these transformations are *similarity transformations* that do not change the structure of the MDS configurations. Differences between two configurations[3] that can be eliminated by similarity transformations cannot possibly be meaningful, because they are *not caused by the data*. We do apply this method for the East and West German MDS configurations using these commands:

```
1   labels.short <- c("interesting","independent","responsibility","meaningful",
2   "advancement","recognition","help others","useful","social","secure job",
3   "income", "spare time", "healthy")
4   attr(EW_eng$west, "Labels") <- attr(EW_eng$east, "Labels") <- labels.short
5   res.west <- mds(sim2diss(EW_eng$west, method="corr"), type="ordinal")
6   res.east <- mds(sim2diss(EW_eng$east, method="corr"), type="ordinal",
7   init=res.west$conf) ## note the initial configuration here
8   fit2 <- Procrustes(res.west$conf, res.east$conf)
9   plot(fit2)
10  ## compute overall similarity measures: r and c
11  r <- cor(as.vector(res.west$conf), as.vector(fit2$Yhat))
12  c <- fit2$congcoef ## congruence coefficient on distances
```

diss <- sim2diss(kipt, method="corr") is doing—is a slightly nonlinear function. This is irrelevant for ordinal MDS, but it shows up in interval MDS.

[3]Procrustean fittings can also be used for configurations that differ in the number of points and in their dimensionalities. For example, the configuration in Fig. 2.13 was fitted to the configuration in Fig. 2.12 to make comparisons easier. The target **X** was derived from Fig. 2.12 by roughly reading off the *X*- and *Y*-coordinates of the centroids of the various value groups. In case of different dimensionalities, one can simply add column vectors with only zeroes to **X** or to **Y**.

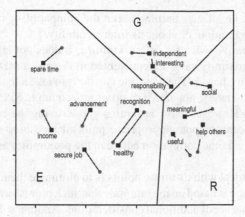

Fig. 7.4 Overlay plot of West German (squares) and East German (dots) work value configurations, optimally matched, with partition based on the ERG theory

The plot in Fig. 7.4 shows the East and the West German results, optimally fitted to each other in one overlay plot. To measure the similarity of the configurations, one can compute the congruence coefficient of corresponding distances ($c = .964$) or the correlation of the coordinates of corresponding points (after Procrustean fitting: $r = .914$). These coefficients can be evaluated against the fit of random configurations (see R script below which yields benchmark values of .88 and .62 for the c- and the r-coefficients, respectively). Hence, the similarity of the observed configurations is much higher than can reasonably be expected by chance.

```
1  Procrustes.test <- function(n,m,nrep=500) { set.seed(333); c <- vector()
2  r <- vector(); X <- matrix(runif(n*m, -1, 1), nrow=n,ncol=m)
3  X <- scale(X, scale=FALSE)
4  for (i in 1:nrep) { Y <- matrix(runif(n*m, -1, 1), nrow=n, ncol=m)
5  fit <- Procrustes(X, Y); c[i] <- fit$congcoef
6  r[i] <- cor(c(X), c(fit$Yhat))}
7  cr <- list("c"=c, "r"=r) }; z <- Procrustes.test(13,2) ## 13 points in 2d
8  z99 <- quantile(z$c, .99); r99 <- quantile(z$r, .99) ## 99% quantiles
9  cat("c(99%)=", round(z99,2), " r(99%)=", round(r99,2), sep = '')
```

Apart from their significant point-to-point similarity, one here notes that both configurations can be partitioned in the same way by Alderfer's E(xistence), R(elations), and G(rowth) theory (Alderfer 1972a). This is a higher-order form of similarity, and it may hold even if the point-wise correspondence is not that high.

7.7 Evaluating Stress Blindly

A frequent mistake of MDS users is that they are often too quick in rejecting an MDS solution because its Stress seems too high. The Stress value is, however, merely a *technical* index, a target criterion for an optimization algorithm. An MDS solution can be robust and replicable, even if its Stress value is high. Stress, moreover, is *substantively blind*; i.e., it says nothing about the compatibility of a content theory with the MDS configuration, or about its interpretability.

Stress is a *summative* index for *all* proximities. It does not inform the user how well a *particular* proximity value is represented in the given MDS space. This was discussed in detail in Chap. 3. The least one can do is to take a look at the Stress-per-point values. Unfortunately, not all MDS programs compute SPP values (or similar point-fit measures). However, most programs allow saving the configuration's distances so that one can compute appropriate point-fit measures with standard data analysis programs (e.g., the correlation between the proximities and the corresponding MDS distances).

A simple way to deal with ill-fitting points is to eliminate them from the analysis. This popular approach is based on the rationale that such points have a special relation to the other points that needs additional considerations. Another solution is to increase the dimensionality of the space so that these points can move into the extra space and form new distances. The rationale in this case is that the proximity of the objects represented by these points to the other points is based on additional dimensions that are not relevant in other comparisons. Experience shows, though, that SPP values are often quite unstable. For example, SPP plots change a lot under different MDS models so that "special" points cannot always be identified with confidence.

In any case, accepting or rejecting an MDS representation on the basis of overall Stress can be too simple. This is easy to see from an example. Consider the West German MDS configuration in Fig. 7.4. If we increase the dimensionality of this solution to $m = 3$, the Stress goes down from 0.17 to 0.09. If we proceed in the same way in case of Fig. 2.2, we get the same reduction in Stress. However, in the former case, the reduction in Stress is caused by essentially two points only. That is, "healthy working conditions" and, in particular, "(much) spare time" clearly move out of the plane in Fig. 7.4 into the third dimension. In case of the country similarity data, all points jitter (some more, some less) about the plane, which looks as if the third dimension is capturing essentially only noise.

For data with large noise components, therefore, low-dimensional MDS solutions can have high Stress values, but they may still be better in terms of theory and replicability than higher-dimensional solutions with lower Stress values. In that case, a low-dimensional solution may be an effective data smoother that brings out the true structure of the data more clearly than an over-fitted high-dimensional MDS representation.

7.8 Always Interpreting Principal Axes Dimensions

Interpreting an MDS solution can be understood as projecting given or conjectured content knowledge onto the MDS configuration. The country similarity example of Sect. 2.2 demonstrates how this is typically done: What one interprets are *dimensions*. MDS users often *automatically* ask for the meaning of "the" dimensions, by which they often mean the axes of the plot that the MDS program delivers. These axes are almost always the principal axes of the solution space. Yet, this dimension system can be arbitrarily rotated and reflected, and oblique dimensions would also span the plane. Hence, users do not have to interpret the dimensions offered by the MDS program, but they could look for m dimensions (in m-dimensional space) that are more meaningful.

There is, however, no natural law that guarantees that dimensions are meaningful at all. Thus, one should be open for other ways of interpreting MDS solutions. One possibility is to look for meaningful *directions* rather than for dimensions. A direction corresponds to a simple line that runs through the MDS plot. When projecting the points of the configuration onto such a line, it becomes an *internal scale*. One can plot such internal scales through a common point such as the centroid of the configuration. Points to the left of this anchor point are given negative scale values; those to the right of it receive positive values. To interpret the internal scale, one studies the point distribution with a focus on content questions such as these: What points lie at the extremes of the scale? How do they differ in terms of content? What is the attribute where they differ most? Why are the points i, j, ... so close together? What do they have in common? Answering such questions gives meaning to the scale.

Additional data can be helpful in such interpretations. We show this for the country similarity example. Table 2.1 exhibits the coordinates of the MDS solution in Fig. 2.2 and the countries' values on two *external* scales, economic development, and number of inhabitants. These scales can be fitted into the MDS space by using the mdsbiplot() function as follows, yielding Fig. 7.5. The fit of the external scales in this MDS configuration is given by the correlation of these scales with the projections of the points onto straight lines through the arrows that represent them. We here get $r = .94$ for economic development and $r = .46$ for the number of inhabitants. (The length of the two arrows represents, approximately, the relative fit of the external scales.) This suggests to interpret this solution in terms of a rotated set of dimensions that correspond to the two arrows representing economic development and number of inhabitants.

```
1  diss <- sim2diss(wish, method=7)
2  res <- mds(diss, type="ordinal")
3  ecdev <- c(3,1,3,3,8,3,7,9,4,7,10,6)
4  inhabs <- c(87,17,8,30,51,500,3,100,750,235,201,20)
5  labs <- attr(wish, "Labels")
6  fitbi <- biplotmds(res, cbind(ecdev, inhabs))
7  plot(fitbi, main="", xlab="", ylab="", cex=1.3,
8       label.conf=list(cex=1.2, pos=ifelse(labs!="RUSSIA", 3, 1)),
9       vecscale=0.5, vec.conf=list(cex=1.2, col="red", cex=1.2, length=0.1))
```

External scales can also help in choosing among different MDS solutions with almost the same Stress. For the country similarity data, ordinal MDS starting with different random configurations leads to a set of different solutions (see Fig. 7.1). Many of them have unacceptably high Stress, but there are different solutions (e.g., #1 and #13) with the same minimal Stress of .185. Figure 7.6 shows these solutions next to each other. In each solution, the two external scales were fitted into the configurations by multiple regression (as in Fig. 2.16, for example).

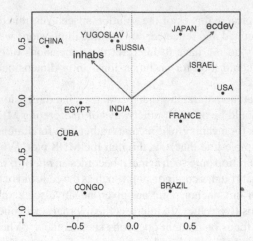

Fig. 7.5 MDS solution for country similarity data; fitted external scales shown as arrows

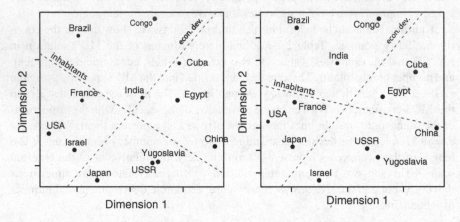

Fig. 7.6 Two same-Stress MDS solutions for country similarity data, with fitted external scales

The two solutions are rather similar (after Procrustean fitting) but differ in two important details: In the left configuration, the positions of Japan and Israel are swapped in comparison with where they are in the right configuration; moreover, in the left configuration, India is positioned more in the center of the configuration. This means that in the configuration on the left, the very large countries are closer together on the line "inhabitants." So, this internal scale correlates with the external scale "number of inhabitants" (see Table 2.1) with $r = .46$ in the left configuration, but only with $r = .30$ in the right configuration. At the same time, the fitted external scales correlate with $r = .93$ in both plots. Hence, the configuration on the left is the somewhat more meaningful MDS solution if one wants to follow Wish (1971) in interpreting the configuration in terms of these dimensions. However, this solution may not be the one that is reported by the MDS program as the final solution, but you can find it if you use a proper initial configuration identified by `icExplore()`.

7.9 Always Interpreting Dimensions or Directions

Dimensions and, more generally, directions are but special cases of *regions*. Regions are subsets of points of an MDS space that are *connected* (i.e., each pair of points in a region can be joined by a curve whose points lie completely within this region), *non-overlapping*, and *exhaustive* (i.e., each point lies in exactly one region). When interpreting MDS solutions, we ask to what extent certain classifications of the objects on the basis of *content facets* correspond to regions of the MDS space. Expressed differently, we ask whether the MDS configuration can be *partitioned* into substantively meaningful regions and, if so, how these regions can be described.

An example for such a partitioning is shown in Fig. 7.4. Here, the different objects ("work values") were first classified into three categories on the basis of a theory by Alderfer (1972b): Work values related to outcomes that satisfy existential-material needs (E), social-relational needs (R), or cognitive-growth needs (G). This ERG typology surfaces in MDS space in certain neighborhoods that can be separated from each other by cutting the plane in a wedge-like fashion. The same type of partitioning is possible both in the West German and also in the East German MDS plane. Hence, the two solutions are equivalent in the ERG sense (Borg and Braun 1996).

Partitioning an MDS space is done *facet by facet*. For each facet F_i, one generates a *facet diagram*. This is simply a copy of the MDS configuration where each point is replaced by the code that indicates to which category of F_i the respective point belongs. One then checks to what extent and in which way this facet diagram can be partitioned into regions that contain only codes of one particular type. The emerging regions should be as simple as possible, e.g. with straight partitioning lines. This is desirable because simple partitions can also be characterized by simple laws of formation that promise to be more robust and more replicable than complicated patterns that are fitted too closely to the particular data and its noise.

Although there exist computer programs that yield partitions for facet diagrams that are optimal in some sense (Borg and Shye 1995), it is typically more fruitful for the user to work with pencil and eraser on a printout of the facet diagram. This way, partitioning lines can be drawn, redrawn, and simplified in an open-eyed fashion, paying attention to content and substantive theory. One may decide, for example, to admit some placements of points in "wrong" regions, because simple overall patterns with some errors are better than perfect partitions with overly complicated partitions.

Three prototypical regionalities that often arise in practice are shown in Fig. 7.7: *axial*, *modular*, and *polar* partitions. Axial and modular partitions are either based on ordered facets, or they suggest ordered facets. Polar partitions, in contrast, are typically related to unordered (nominal) facets. Of course, if the sectors in a polar partition are arranged similarly in many replications, then one should think about reasons for this order.

Regionalizations—simple ones, in particular—become unlikely to result by chance if the number of points goes up. That is easy to see from a thought experiment. Assume you take a set of n ping-pong balls and label some of them with "a", others

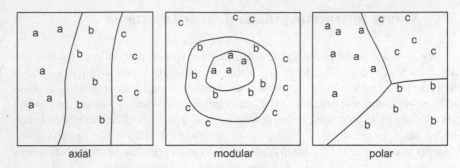

Fig. 7.7 Prototypical partitioning of MDS configurations by three facets, each one with three categories (a, b, c)

with "b", and still others with "c". Then, throw them all into a bucket, mix them thoroughly, and pour the bucket onto the floor. After the balls come to their parking positions, try to partition the resulting configuration into a-, b-, and c-regions. This will be difficult or even impossible if you want simple regions as in Fig. 7.7. It is even less likely that the regionality that you find in one case can be replicated when the experiment is repeated. A simple regional pattern, therefore, suggests a lawful relationship in the sense that *the facet structures the observations*. This notion becomes even more powerful if an MDS configuration can be partitioned by more than one facet so that the different organizational patterns can be stacked on top of each other as, for example, in the radex in Fig. 2.8.

An MDS solution can be partitioned, in principle, by as many facets as the user can think of. There is no fixed relation between the number of facets and the dimensionality of the space. This is different for dimensions: In an m-dimensional space, one always seeks to interpret exactly m dimensions. A dimensional interpretation corresponds to a combination of m axial facets (see Fig. 7.7, left panel), each generating an ordered set of (infinitely) narrow bands with linear boundary lines so that a grid-like mesh (as, e.g., in Fig. 6.3) is generated.

Regions are sometimes confused with *clusters*. Clusters, however, are but special cases of regions. They are often defined as lumps (or chains) of points surrounded by empty space so that each point in a cluster is always closer to at least one point in the cluster than to any point not in the cluster. Clustering in that sense is not required for perfect regions. Regions are like countries that cut a continent like Europe into pieces. Malmö/Sweden, for example, is much closer to Copenhagen/Denmark—both are connected by a bridge—than to any other Swedish city, so the Swedish cities do not form a cluster on the European map, but they are all in the same region.

Clusters, moreover, are *formal* constructs, while regions are based on *substantive* thinking that is often expressed via facets. Nevertheless, one can always cluster proximities and then check how the resulting clusters organize the points of an MDS solution. Cluster analysis is, however, not particularly robust: Different amalgamation criteria can lead to vastly different clusters. Cluster analysis, therefore, is not a method for "validating" an MDS solution or interpretation, as some writers argue.

Rather, cluster analysis typically just leads to groupings of points that tend to surface similarly in MDS solutions.

7.10   Poorly Dealing with Disturbing Points

A frequent problem in MDS applications is what to do with points that do not fit into an interpretation. A typical case is a configuration that cannot be partitioned in a theoretically pleasing way because of one or a few "misplaced" points. In such cases, one may decide to construct (slightly) overlapping regions, or stick to the partitioning notion and generate curvy partitioning lines (as, e.g., in Fig. 6.2). A third solution is to draw a best-possible partitioning system where some points remain in regions to which they do not belong. A fourth, and often rather dubious solution, is to eliminate such points from the MDS configuration by "explaining them away" in substantive terms.

A completely different way to deal with disturbing points is asking how much the Stress goes up if one shifts these points in space such that simple partitioning becomes possible. The easiest way to answer this question is the following. Assume you use `res <- mds(diss, type="interval")`. Now, replace the coordinates of disturbing points in `res$conf` with "should" coordinates (i.e., coordinates that put these points into positions where they are not disturbing anymore). Let us call this modified coordinate matrix `X.mod`. Then, compute the Stress of `X.mod` using the `stress0()` function: `stress0(diss, init=X.mod, type="interval")`. Finally, compare the Stress value of the optimal solution `res$conf` with the Stress of `X.mod`. If the Stress increment is small, then one would probably prefer the solution that allows a simple interpretation over the optimal-Stress solution. The rationale is that it promises to be better replicable, being based on a substantive law of formation, than the solution that represents the one given set of data with minimal Stress.

A formally better solution is using confirmatory MDS. However, confirmatory MDS with regional restrictions can be difficult to formulate and to implement. Hence, before trying this, a simple shift-and-see approach yields a quick answer that is often sufficient. Note, though, that replications are *absolutely essential* in any case. If certain disturbing points come out similarly in replications, one must take a closer look at what exactly is being measured by them and how this is related to the rest of the variables. A small increment in global Stress when shifting a few points can also be *deceptive*, in particular if only one or two points are moved and the rest of a large configuration is not changed. A vivid example is the case of the Morse signals in Fig. 6.3, where only one point (the signal for "1") is substantially shifted out of a total of 36 points. This one-point movement cannot affect the Stress very much and so this one signal remains suspicious.

7.11 Scaling Almost-Equal Proximities

Proximity data cannot always be represented in a low-dimensional space. This is true, for example, if the data have a large error component or if they are simply random data. A second instance is data that are essentially constant. Buja et al. (1994) have shown that if all data are exactly equal, 2d ratio MDS leads to points that all lie on concentric circles; moreover, the points can all be interchanged without affecting the Stress. Users should therefore keep an eye on the case of almost-equal proximities or disparities. In particular, they must look closely at the units of the Y-axis of the Shepard diagram: If most of these values are almost equal, then caution is needed. Most computer programs choose an origin for the Y axis that magnifies the range of the observed values. If the origin of Y in a Shepard plot is zero, then the almost-equal problem becomes obvious immediately. Also, investigate the distribution of the proximities or disparities, preferably in a histogram. If the histogram shows that the disparities are all close together and are much different from zero, then one can expect the 2d solution of concentric circles.

Another way to diagnose peculiarities in the data is scaling them with different MDS models. In case of almost-equal proximities, ordinal MDS preserving ties (secondary approach) and interval MDS yield almost the same results. However, if ordinal MDS is used with the primary approach to ties—which allows to untie ties in the distances—a radically different solution is obtained, where most of the points cluster in one point, and a few points scatter about this cluster. The Stress, moreover, is much smaller than for the other MDS representations. If different MDS models yield such vastly different results, then something is almost always wrong. With well-structured data, different MDS models yield solutions that do not differ much.

7.12 Summary

Some mistakes are frequently made in MDS. One example is not specifying the proper polarity of proximities so that the MDS program uses similarity data as dis-similarity data, or vice versa. Another simple mistake is making MDS programs terminate their iterations too early, or not studying the effects of using different starting configurations. Once aware of these mistakes, they can be easily avoided. Another mistake is overlooking degenerate solutions in ordinal MDS. They can be avoided by using stronger MDS models. A rather frequent mistake is automatically asking for the meaning of "the" dimensions: Dimensions are but a special case of regions, and other meaningful patterns may also exist in an MDS configuration. Simply discarding disturbing points from an MDS solution is also too mechanical: Sometimes, such points can be shifted without affecting the Stress very much. Then, when comparing different MDS solutions, one should first get rid of meaningless differences via Procrustean transformations. Finally, data that are almost all equal can lead to meaningless MDS solutions.

References

Alderfer, C. P. (1972a). *Existence, relatedness, and growth*. New York: Free Press.

Alderfer, C. P. (1972b). *Existence, relatedness, and growth*. New York: Free Press.

Borg, I., & Braun, M. (1996). Work values in East and West Germany: Different weights but identical structures. *Journal of Organizational Behavior*, *17*, 541–555.

Borg, I., & Mair, P. (2017). The choice of initial configurations in multidimensional scaling: local minima, fit, and interpretability. *Austrian Journal of Statistics*, *46*, 19–32.

Borg, I., & Shye, S. (1995). *Facet theory: Form and content*. Newbury Park, CA: Sage.

Buja, A., Logan, B. F., Reeds, J. R., & Shepp, L. A. (1994). Inequalities and positive-definite functions arising from a problem in multidimensional scaling. *The Annals of Statistics*, *22*, 406–438.

Guthrie, J. T. (1973). Models of reading and reading disability. *Journal of Educational Psychology*, *65* 9–18.

Wish, M. (1971). Individual differences in perceptions and preferences among nations. In C. W. King & D. Tigert (Eds.), *Attitude research reaches new heights* (pp. 312–328). Chicago: American Marketing Association.

References

...

Chapter 8
Unfolding

Abstract Unfolding is discussed again in a realistic and more complex application that requires a 3d solution with a special rotation. For mixed samples, multidimensional unfolding can sometimes be replaced by multiple low-dimensional unfolding. One must also clarify whether the data are unconditionally comparable. The stability of unfolding solutions is discussed, and some special unfolding models such as the vector model and circular unfolding are introduced.

Keywords Unfolding · External unfolding · Internal unfolding
Conditionalities · Vector model unfolding · Circular unfolding

8.1 Unfolding in Three-Dimensional Space

To discuss the various issues involved in three-dimensional (3d) unfolding, we use the PVQ40 data set, but now we scale value indexes based on the observed ("raw") ratings, not on centered ratings. To turn the preference indexes into dissimilarity indexes, we first subtract the observed importance ratings from the maximum rating value. This leads to a dissimilarity value of zero for those persons who fully endorse a value. The dissimilarities are then scaled using the unfolding() function of the SMACOF package (see R script below[1]).

The 3d ratio scale unfolding solution is shown in Fig. 8.1. It has a Stress of 0.205, indicating a good fit of the 151×10 data matrix to the corresponding 1,510 distances in unfolding space. The permutation test of unfolding() finds that this Stress value has a p-value smaller than 0.01. Hence, the solution is "significant."

---

[1]Note that you can use this script and hold the s2 matrix of the initial configuration fixed if you want to do external unfolding with a theory-derived configuration of value points. To do this, you add the argument fix = "columns" to the unfolding() call.

© The Author(s) 2018
I. Borg et al., *Applied Multidimensional Scaling and Unfolding*,
SpringerBriefs in Statistics, https://doi.org/10.1007/978-3-319-73471-2_8

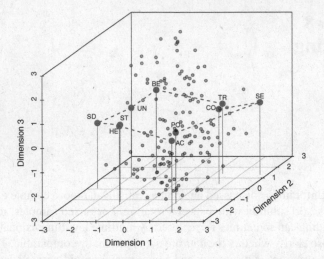

Fig. 8.1 Unfolding configuration of importance ratings on personal values (reversed, subtracted from max scale value); person points unlabeled; value points marked as PO, AC, ... , SE and connected in the order of the Schwartz value circle

The configuration in Fig. 8.1 has been rotated to an orientation where the first two dimensions coincide with the first two principal axes of the points representing the ten basic values. This is accomplished as follows. Let $\mathbf{X}$ be the coordinate matrix of the value points and $\mathbf{Y}$ the coordinates of the person points. We compute the singular value decomposition $\mathbf{X} = \mathbf{PDQ}'$ and then use $\mathbf{Q}$ to rotate $\mathbf{X}$ and $\mathbf{Y}$ to $\mathbf{XQ}$ and $\mathbf{YQ}$, respectively. $\mathbf{XQ}$ yields a principal axes orientation of $\mathbf{X}$, because $\mathbf{XQ} = \mathbf{PD}$ has orthogonal columns of maximal norm (Borg and Groenen 2005, p. 162).

Scaling solutions in 3d space are difficult to interpret. Most programs offer graphical output in the form of three planes, i.e., the planes spanned by the configuration's principal axes. Inspecting these planes does not always guarantee seeing the substantive meaning of the configuration. In the given case, the principal axes orientation of the 3d unfolding configuration is substantively inaccessible. In such a case, it can be helpful to use *interactive* graphics that allow rotating the configuration in space to orientations that are more revealing. For example, in the R environment, one can interactively study the configuration of the points representing the personal values with coordinate matrix $\mathbf{X}$ by using `library(rgl); plot3d(X, size = 10);` `text3d(X, text = colnames(PVQ40agg), adj = 1.2)` and save the plot[2] with `rgl.postscript("myplot.pdf", fmt = "pdf")`.

---

[2]For more information, see http://www.sthda.com/english/wiki/a-complete-guide-to-3d-visualization-device-system-in-r-r-software-and-data-visualization.

```
 1 nobs <- dim(PVQ40agg)[1]
 2 set.seed(33) ## sets a seed for the random number generator
 3 ## Initial configuration of personal values (based on TUV theory)
 4 tuv <- matrix(c(.50,-.87,.71,-.71,.87,-.50,.87,.50,.50,.87,-.50,.87,
 5          -.71,.71,-.87,.50,-.87,-.50,-.50,-.87), nrow=10, ncol=2, byrow=TRUE)
 6 s2 <- cbind(tuv, matrix(0, nrow=10, ncol=1)) ## Add column of zeros for 3d
 7 ## Initial configuration of persons (random)
 8 s1 <- matrix(runif(3*nobs, min=0, max=1), nrow=nobs, ncol=3)
 9 pref <- max(PVQ40agg) - PVQ40agg  ## Preferences into dissimilarities
10 result <- unfolding(delta=pref, ndim=3, itmax=6000, init=list(s1, s2))
11 result; permtest(result)
12 e <- svd(result$conf.col)
13 X <- result$conf.col %*% e$v  # Rotation to principal axes
14 eV <- sum(X[, 1:2]^2) / sum(X^2) # expl.var. in value plane
15 Y <- result$conf.row %*% e$v # Rotation to principal axes
16 ## plot 3d unfolding solution --------------------------------------------
17 require(scatterplot3d)
18 lim1 <- c(-3,+3)
19 s3d <- scatterplot3d(X, type="h", xlab="Dimension 1", ylab="Dimension 2",
20                     zlab="Dimension 3", xlim=lim1, ylim=lim1, zlim=lim1,
21                     cex.symbols=2,color="red", pch=21, bg="red", asp=1)
22 text(s3d$xyz.convert(X), labels=colnames(raw), pos=3 )
23 s3d$points3d(rbind(X, X[1, ]), type="l", col="blue", lty=2, lwd=2)
24 s3d$points3d(Y, pch=21, bg=grey(0.1, alpha=.4),
25             col-grey(0.1, alpha=.6), xlab="", ylab="")
26 plot(result, plot.type="stressplot") ## plot SPPs persons/values
```

Unfolding in only two dimensions generates a solution that is uninterpretable. The value circle, in particular, does not emerge at all in this solution. For the 3d configuration in Fig. 8.1, one finds that the value points are almost fully contained in the 1–2 plane of the rotated configuration: The plane captures 97.4% of the value points' variance in the 3d unfolding space. One also notes in Fig. 8.1 that the value points are almost perfectly ordered as predicted by Schwartz (1992). This becomes even clearer when looking at this space from above along the third dimension (Fig. 8.2).

The configuration of the value points in the 1–2 plane is also quite similar to the configuration of the value points in the 2d unfolding solution for centered ratings shown in Fig. 2.14: After Procrustean fitting, the corresponding point coordinates correlate with $r = 0.96$. Moreover, the perpendicular distances of the person points from the 1–2 plane of the value points correlate with the corresponding mean ratings of the persons with $r = -0.84$. Thus, persons with high mean value ratings are close to the plane of the value circle, and persons with low mean ratings are far away from this plane.

Figure 8.3 gives the SPP distributions of the various persons and the 10 value points, respectively. In the plot on the left-hand side, one notes that person #21 has the worst fit in the unfolding space. This person has scores of 6.0 for AC and CO; 4.0 for TR; 3.5 for PO; 2.7 for UN; 2.0 for SE; 1.5 for ST; and 1.0 for HE, SD, and BE. Hence, he/she should be located close to AC and CO in unfolding space, but this would automatically put him/her very close to PO and close to SE (see Fig. 8.2), and that would not represent his/her importance ratings so well. On the other hand, if this person is located somewhere in this neighborhood, then his/her distances to the points BE, HE, and SD are large, and this expresses his/her ratings properly.

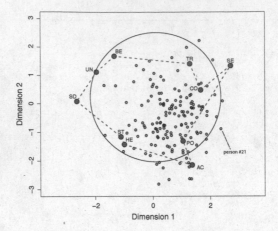

Fig. 8.2 Plane spanned by Dimension 1 and 2 of Fig. 8.1; points connected as predicted by Schwartz's theory; circle optimally fitted to value points

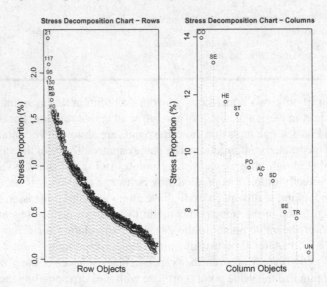

Fig. 8.3 SPP values for persons (left) and for personal values (right) in unfolding solution in Fig. 8.1

Hence, even this person fits reasonably well into the unfolding solution. The best compromise position found by unfolding for person #21 is shown in Fig. 8.2.

8.2 Multidimensional Versus Multiple Unfolding

Assume that we have a data set of preferences of various persons for different political parties. A typical way to think about such data is to assume that these persons all perceive the parties similarly in terms of their left-to-right orientation. That is, the Communist party is on the far left, the Nationalists on the far right. The persons differ, however, in their political preferences. This is the classical unfolding scenario: The closer a party to the ideal point of a person, the stronger this person's preference for this party. Hence, unfolding the observed ratings or rankings should lead to a one-dimensional solution of person and party points. It may, therefore, come as a surprise that Norpoth (1979) reports that representative data sets of potential voters rank-ordering major political parties in Germany cannot be scaled in one dimension. Rather, the solution spaces are two-dimensional.

As a psychological model of preference, the unfolding model rests on a rather strong assumption: All persons share the *same perception* of the objects. What if this assumption is wrong? Reanalyzing the above voter preferences, Borg and Staufenbiel (2007) showed that some voters located the German Liberals to the right of the Conservatives, while other voters swapped the order of these parties. If the two groups of voters are thrown into one single unfolding analysis, a hard-to-interpret two-dimensional solution is needed to represent these data. If, however, the two groups are analyzed separately (*multiple unfolding*), unfolding leads to a 1d solution for each group, where the Liberals are to the left of the Conservatives in one data set, and to the right in the other. Thus, the multidimensional unfolding representation for the total sample appears to be an aggregation artifact that does not properly represent the preferential space of normal voters.

Another feature of the unfolding model is that the preference strength of each person should drop monotonically as a function of the distance from his/her ideal point. Now consider the case where persons are asked to rank-order different samples of tea that differ in their temperature, from steaming hot to ice cold. One can assume here that the persons will produce preference ratings that cannot be unfolded in one dimension. Yet, multidimensionality would be the wrong way out in this case too. Rather, what we have here are two essentially incomparable types of objects, hot tea and iced tea, and the ratings for each of them should be scaled separately in 1d space.

8.3 Conditionalities in Unfolding

In unfolding, one should consider whether one really wants to assume that the data are comparable across rows. In our example on preferences for personal values, one may doubt that an importance rating of "4", say, of person i is truly equal to the "4" given by person j. Some persons use high scores throughout, others shy away from extreme scores. Social desirability, acquiescence, and other response style artifacts may also affect the ratings. This is why such data are often centered, person by person. But even then, the cautious researcher may not want to compare the data across individuals. This means, he/she wants to *split the data matrix by rows* and use a person-specific regression for each single row of the data matrix. Thus, for example, in ratio unfolding, this *row-conditional* treatment of the data allows a specific multiplicative constant *for each individual*. This would lead to a Shepard diagram with as many regression lines as there are persons. In the matrix-conditional case in Fig. 3.4, we have only one regression line—the same for all persons.

Such conditionalities may be desirable for theoretical reasons. However, they further reduce what is already scarce in unfolding, i.e., the constraints that the data exert onto the distances of the solution. For row-conditional unfolding, one should, therefore, have "plenty" of data (rule of thumb: at least 15 persons, all with different preference profiles).

In general, we do not recommend beginning an unfolding analysis of preference data with weak models (e.g., ordinal unfolding with row conditionality). Rather, begin with the *opposite* as in the example above in Sect. 8.1, i.e., a strong model such as ratio unconditional unfolding. This takes the data seriously, allowing no admissible transformations but mapping each observed score directly into a model distance. A weaker model should only be tested if the stronger model cannot be salvaged.

8.4   Stability of Unfolding Solutions

From a geometric point of view, unfolding can easily lead to unstable solutions. This is so because the model rests on data that constrain only a subset of the distances, namely the distances between ideal points and object points, but not the distances among ideal points and also not the distances among object points (see Table 1.2b).

Moreover, with real data, object points and ideal points are often not thoroughly mixed. That is, many preference orders that are theoretically possible do not appear at all, because most persons prefer or reject the same objects. This can lead to major indeterminacies of the unfolding solution, where single points can be moved around arbitrarily in ample solution regions without affecting the Stress (see Borg and Groenen 2005).

You can test the stability of unfolding by choosing different seeds in the R commands above. Simply replace the 33 in set.seed(33) by 1, 47, or any other number. These seeds lead to different random components in the initial configuration, and this can lead to different solutions. For applied research, this means that you would hope to eventually find a solution that is theoretically convincing *and* that has an acceptable Stress value (if it exists). It sometimes pays to test different starting configurations and then pick the solution with the most desirable properties (see also p. 78f.).

8.5   Degenerate Unfolding Solutions

A major problem in unfolding is the risk to obtain degenerate solutions, in particular when using weak unfolding models. The solutions, then, show peculiar patterns where all distances between ideal points and object points are essentially equal. Such undesirable solutions are sometimes easily recognized, for example, if the person points are all located on a circular arc, while the object points are lumped together in the center of the circle. To avoid this problem, most unfolding programs use slightly modified target functions when searching for an optimal solution, but they are often not successful. A systematic approach that avoids degenerate solutions was proposed by Busing et al. (2005) and implemented in the PREFSCAL module of SPSS and in `unfolding()` in SMACOF. It penalizes the loss function whenever the MDS configuration tends to be modified in the optimization process into the direction of equal distances. We, therefore, recommend using these programs in case of interval and ordinal unfolding.

Another issue is weighting the rows of the data matrix. In case of the PVQ40 ratings of importance of personal values, some persons generate highly different ratings, others rate all values the same. The latter data are easy to represent in unfolding in a quasi-degenerate solution with the person points densely clustered in the center of a circle of points representing the personal values. So, if you have a large proportion of persons with almost constant ratings, unfolding becomes almost trivial. To counteract this tendency toward a trivial solution, one can weight the data somehow by their variance. Assume that `pref` are the preferences converted to dissimilarities (as on p. 97), then these commands are one possibility in SMACOF:

```
1 pref <- max(PVQ40agg) - PVQ40agg; nper <- dim(pref)[1]
2 var.per.row <- apply(pref, 1, var)
3 W <- matrix(var.per.row, nrow = nper, ncol = ncol(pref))
4 W[W==0] <- min( W[W!=min(W)] ) ## if var=0, use smallest non-zero variance
5 out <- unfolding(pref, weightmat = W)
```

8.6 Special Unfolding Models

Three special unfolding models are worth mentioning. One is *weighted unfolding*. It assumes that all persons share a common perception of the choice objects, but now each person can also take the common space and stretch it differentially along its dimensions (or along idiosyncratically rotated dimensions) before placing an ideal point into this space. An even more general model admits negative dimension weights and anti-ideal points (Carroll, 1980). Practical applications show, however, that little is gained by going beyond the simple unfolding model. Moreover, some of these (extremely complicated) models turn out to have obscure properties when looking more closely. Hence, weighted unfolding is not recommended for the applied user.

Another case is the *vector model* of unfolding. It represents the persons by *directed lines* running through the origin, not by ideal points. Each such line is oriented in space such that the projections of the points representing the choice objects onto this line correspond optimally to the observed preference scores of a person. Expressed differently, each person's preference scores are explained by a weighted sum of the dimensions of the objects. For example, person p may weight Dimension 1 by 60%

Fig. 8.4 Vector model
unfolding of basic value
index scores of 151 persons;
each arrow represents a
person; person 133 marked
by a line; arrow shows
direction and strength of
persons' strivings in value
space

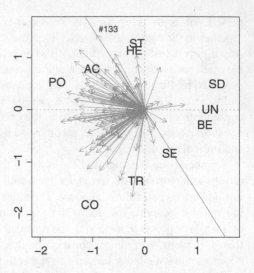

and Dimension 2 by 40% and give both a positive sign (more=better). This defines
the orientation of p's preference vector: It runs into the 2:00 o'clock direction.[3]

Figure 8.4 shows a 2d solution of a linear version of this model for the PVQ40 data.
Each arrow in the plot represents a different person. An arrow shows the direction
and the resultant strength of a person's striving in value space. Computationally, we
get this plot from the following R script:

```
1  vmu -<- function (P, ndim=2, center=TRUE, scale=FALSE) {
2    m <- dim(P)[2]; S <- svd(t(scale(t(P), center=center, scale=scale)))
3    X <- m^(1/2)*S$v; Y <- m^(-1/2)*S$u %*% diag(S$d)  ## X=objects, Y=persons
4    row.names(X) <- colnames(P); row.names(Y) <- rownames(P)
5    return(list(X=X[,1:ndim], Y=Y[,1:ndim], VAF=sum(S$d[1:ndim]^2)/sum(S$d^2),
6    d=S$d))- }
7  res <- vmu(PVQ40agg)   ## calling function vmu with PVQ40agg data
8  plot(1.2*res$X[,1], 1.2*res$X[,2], type="n", asp=1, xlab="", ylab="")
9  abline(0, res$Y[133,2]/res$Y[133,1], col="gray"); abline(h=0, v=0, lty=2)
10 zero <- rep(0,nrow(res$Y))
11 arrows(zero, zero, res$Y[,1], res$Y[,2], col="red", length=0.1)  ## persons
12 text(res$X[,1], res$X[,2], rownames(res$X), cex=1.5)  ## objects
13 text(res$Y[133,1], res$Y[133,2], labels="133")
14 round(PVQ40agg[133,],2); round(PVQ40agg[133,]-mean(PVQ40agg[133,]),2)
15 round(t(res$X %*% res$Y[133,]), 2)  ## reconstructed values of person 133
16 round(t(res$X %*% res$Y[133,]/(sum(res$Y[133,]^2)^.5)),2)  ## projected values
```

Overall, the solution accounts for 66% of the variance. The arrow representing
person #133 is marked by a solid line running from the upper left-hand side of the
plot to the lower right-hand side. It explains this person's data quite well, except for

---

[3]The vector model cannot represent cases where a person's preference strengths keep going up
until a certain point is reached and then drop monotonically as one continues moving further on
the person's vector. If, however, all ideal points move far outside the configuration of the choice
objects, the vector model approximates the ideal-point model as a special case (Coombs, 1975).

some discrepancies on HE and AC. The (centered) ratings of person #133 correlate
with the his/her reconstructed[4] scores with $r = 0.947$:

```
                 SE    CO    TR    BE    UN    SD    ST    HE    AC    PO
value ratings  -1.77 -1.77 -1.77 -1.77 -1.10  0.23  1.73  0.73  3.23  2.23
reconstructed  -1.64 -1.66 -1.81 -1.46 -1.13 -0.53  2.00  1.84  2.07  2.31
```

The unfolding solution shows that most persons in this sample lean toward self-
enhancement, not toward self-transcendence. We also note once more that the object
points form a roughly circular configuration, similar to the ideal-point solution in
Figs. 3.4 and 1.11.

The third special model is *circular* unfolding. This model is the same as regular
ideal-point unfolding, except that it imposes a particular restriction onto the object
points (or the person points): They must all lie on a circle. An application of this
model is the case of importance ratings for personal values. Figure 1.11 shows the
solution of unrestricted unfolding for ten (centered) value indexes and 146 persons
(PVQ40 data). It also shows a circle that was fitted to the configuration of points
that represent the personal values. In circular unfolding, we search for an unfolding
solution where all value points (formally: "column points") are strictly on a circle. To
compute this solution, the user only needs to set one additional argument when calling the unfolding function: `result <- unfolding(pref, circle = "column")`.
This generates a perfect-circle solution with a Stress of .175. Without the circle constraint, we get Fig. 1.11, with a Stress of .167. Obviously, the additional constraint
made almost no difference in terms of the overall model fit, and so this is an attractive
unfolding model, because it suggests a simple law of formation.

8.7   Summary

Unfolding in 3d space leads to special problems. The usual principal axes rotation
may not allow a meaningful interpretation. To rotate the unfolding space, one can
use interactive graphics or theory-driven analytic approaches. The user should know
that unfolding solutions can be too high-dimensional because the samples consist of
subgroups with different common spaces. This can lead to misinterpretations of the
unfolding solution. Also, in unfolding, the user needs to decide if his/her data should
be considered comparable across persons. If they are taken as row-conditionally
comparable only, the unfolding model is weakened, just as assuming ordinal or
interval scale levels. Degenerate solutions are almost certain to result in such cases,
unless special unfolding programs are used that systematically avoid such solutions.
If possible, strong unfolding models or even special unfolding models such as the
vector model or circular unfolding are, therefore, to be preferred.

---

[4]The reconstructed values are obtained by projecting each item onto the direction of the person
arrow multiplied by the length of the person arrow.

References

Borg, I., & Groenen, P. J. F. (2005). *Modern multidimensional scaling* (2nd ed.). New York: Springer.
Borg, I., & Staufenbiel, T. (2007). *Theorien und methoden der skalierung* (4th ed.). Berne: Huber.
Busing, F. M. T. A., Groenen, P. J. F., & Heiser, W. J. (2005). Avoiding degeneracy in multidimensional unfolding by penalizing on the coefficient of variation. *Psychometrika, 70*, 71–98.
Carroll, J. D. (1980). Models and methods for multidimensional analysis of preferential choice or other dominance data. In E. D. Lantermann & H. Feger (Eds.), *Similarity and choice*. Bern: Huber.
Coombs, C. H. (1975). A note on the relation between the vector model and the unfolding model for preferences. *Psychometrika, 40*, 115–116.
Norpoth, H. (1979). The parties come to order! Dimensions of preferential choice in the West German electorate, 1961–1976. *The American Political Science Review, 73*, 724–736.
Schwartz, S. H. (1992). Universals in the content and structure of values: Theoretical advances and empirical tests in 20 countries. *Advances in Experimental Social Psychology, 25*, 1–65.

Chapter 9
MDS Algorithms

Abstract Two types of solutions for MDS are discussed. If the proximities are Euclidean distances, classical MDS yields an easy algebraic solution. In most MDS applications, iterative methods are needed, because they admit many types of data and distances. They use a two-phase optimization algorithm, moving the points in MDS space in small steps while holding the data and their transforms fixed, and vice versa, until convergence is reached.

Keywords Classical MDS · Iterative MDS algorithm · Disparity
Two-phase algorithm · Rational starting configuration · Majorization · SMACOF

For most MDS models, a best-possible solution $\mathbf{X}$ cannot be found by simply solving a system of equations. The conditions for MDS solutions are so complicated, in general, that they are algebraically untractable. MDS solutions must, therefore, be approximated iteratively, using intelligent search procedures (algorithms) that reduce the Stress by repeatedly moving the points somewhat to new locations and by successively rescaling the proximities until a Stress minimum is found.

Algorithms of this kind are not needed if one wants to assume or if one can prove that the dissimilarity data δ_{ij}—possibly derived first from inverting similarity data—are Euclidean distances. In this case, *classical MDS* can be used to find the MDS solution $\mathbf{X}$ analytically.

9.1 Classical MDS

Classical MDS—also known as *Torgerson scaling* and as *Torgerson-Gower scaling*—works as follows:

1. Square the $n \times n$ dissimilarity data: $\mathbf{\Delta}^{(2)}$.

© The Author(s) 2018

I. Borg et al., *Applied Multidimensional Scaling and Unfolding*,
SpringerBriefs in Statistics, https://doi.org/10.1007/978-3-319-73471-2_9

2. Convert the squared dissimilarities to scalar products through double centering[1] of $\mathbf{\Delta}^{(2)}$: $\mathbf{B_\Delta} = -\frac{1}{2}\mathbf{Z}\mathbf{\Delta}^{(2)}\mathbf{Z}$, where $\mathbf{Z} = \mathbf{I} - n^{-1}\mathbf{J}$, and where $\mathbf{I}$ is the identity matrix (with all elements in the main diagonal equal to 1, and all others equal to 0), and $\mathbf{J}$ is a matrix of ones.

3. Compute the eigen-decomposition $\mathbf{B_\Delta} = \mathbf{Q\Lambda Q}'$.

4. Take the first m eigenvalues greater than 0 ($=\mathbf{\Lambda}_+$) and the corresponding first m columns of $\mathbf{Q}$ ($=\mathbf{Q}_+$). The solution of classical MDS is $\mathbf{X} = \mathbf{Q}_+\mathbf{\Lambda}_+^{1/2}$.

We demonstrate these steps with a small numerical example:

$$\mathbf{\Delta} = \begin{bmatrix} 0 & 4.05 & 8.25 & 5.57 \\ 4.05 & 0 & 2.54 & 2.69 \\ 8.25 & 2.54 & 0 & 2.11 \\ 5.57 & 2.69 & 2.11 & 0 \end{bmatrix}, \text{ which leads to } \mathbf{\Delta}^{(2)} = \begin{bmatrix} 0.00 & 16.40 & 68.06 & 31.02 \\ 16.40 & 0.00 & 6.45 & 7.24 \\ 68.06 & 6.45 & 0.00 & 4.45 \\ 31.02 & 7.24 & 4.45 & 0.00 \end{bmatrix}.$$

In the second step, we compute

$$\mathbf{B_\Delta} = -\frac{1}{2}\mathbf{Z}\mathbf{\Delta}^{(2)}\mathbf{Z}$$

$$= -\frac{1}{2}\begin{bmatrix} \frac{3}{4} & -\frac{1}{4} & -\frac{1}{4} & -\frac{1}{4} \\ -\frac{1}{4} & \frac{3}{4} & -\frac{1}{4} & -\frac{1}{4} \\ -\frac{1}{4} & -\frac{1}{4} & \frac{3}{4} & -\frac{1}{4} \\ -\frac{1}{4} & -\frac{1}{4} & -\frac{1}{4} & \frac{3}{4} \end{bmatrix} \begin{bmatrix} 0.00 & 16.40 & 68.06 & 31.02 \\ 16.40 & 0.00 & 6.45 & 7.24 \\ 68.06 & 6.45 & 0.00 & 4.45 \\ 31.02 & 7.24 & 4.45 & 0.00 \end{bmatrix} \begin{bmatrix} \frac{3}{4} & -\frac{1}{4} & -\frac{1}{4} & -\frac{1}{4} \\ -\frac{1}{4} & \frac{3}{4} & -\frac{1}{4} & -\frac{1}{4} \\ -\frac{1}{4} & -\frac{1}{4} & \frac{3}{4} & -\frac{1}{4} \\ -\frac{1}{4} & -\frac{1}{4} & -\frac{1}{4} & \frac{3}{4} \end{bmatrix}$$

$$= \begin{bmatrix} 20.52 & 1.64 & -18.08 & -4.09 \\ 1.64 & -0.83 & 2.05 & -2.87 \\ -18.08 & 2.05 & 11.39 & 4.63 \\ -4.09 & -2.87 & 4.63 & 2.33 \end{bmatrix}.$$

In the third step, we compute the eigen-decomposition of $\mathbf{B_\Delta} = \mathbf{Q\Lambda Q}'$ with

$$\mathbf{Q} = \begin{bmatrix} 0.77 & 0.04 & 0.50 & -0.39 \\ 0.01 & -0.61 & 0.50 & 0.61 \\ -0.61 & -0.19 & 0.50 & -0.59 \\ -0.18 & 0.76 & 0.50 & 0.37 \end{bmatrix} \text{ and } \mathbf{\Lambda} = \begin{bmatrix} 35.71 & 0.00 & 0.00 & 0.00 \\ 0.00 & 3.27 & 0.00 & 0.00 \\ 0.00 & 0.00 & 0.00 & 0.00 \\ 0.00 & 0.00 & 0.00 & -5.57 \end{bmatrix}.$$

In the fourth step, this yields the MDS configuration

$$\mathbf{X} = \mathbf{Q}_+\mathbf{\Lambda}_+^{1/2}$$

$$= \begin{bmatrix} 0.77 & 0.04 \\ 0.01 & -0.61 \\ -0.61 & -0.19 \\ -0.18 & 0.76 \end{bmatrix} \begin{bmatrix} 5.98 & 0.00 \\ 0.00 & 1.81 \end{bmatrix} = \begin{bmatrix} 4.62 & 0.07 \\ 0.09 & -1.11 \\ -3.63 & -0.34 \\ -1.08 & 1.38 \end{bmatrix}.$$

---

[1]This means that the centroid of the MDS configuration becomes the origin. The coordinates of $\mathbf{X}$, thus, should sum to 0 in each column of $\mathbf{X}$. This does not carry any consequences for the distances of $\mathbf{X}$; that is, any other point could also serve as the origin. However, one point must be picked as an origin to compute scalar products.

To check the goodness of this solution, we compare its distances with the given dissimilarities, Δ. The distances are

$$
\mathbf{D} = \begin{bmatrix} 0.00 & 4.68 & 8.26 & 3.60 \\ 4.68 & 0.00 & 5.85 & 2.75 \\ 8.26 & 5.85 & 0.00 & 3.08 \\ 3.80 & 2.75 & 3.08 & 0.00 \end{bmatrix}, \text{ so that } \Delta - \mathbf{D} = \begin{bmatrix} 0.00 & -0.63 & -0.01 & 1.97 \\ -0.63 & 0.00 & -3.31 & -0.06 \\ -0.01 & -3.31 & 0.00 & -0.97 \\ 1.77 & -0.06 & -0.97 & 0.00 \end{bmatrix}.
$$

In this example, the distances among the points of the MDS configuration constructed by classical MDS are only approximately equal to the given dissimilarity data. The reason for this result is that the dissimilarities in Δ are *not* Euclidean distances, as classical MDS assumes. Mathematicians would have noticed that in the third step above, because if the dissimilarities are Euclidean distances, then all eigenvalues are non-negative. If negative eigenvalues occur, one may decide to "explain them away" as caused by "error" in the dissimilarities, provided that these negative eigenvalues are relatively small. In the above example, however, this assumption appears hard to justify, because the one negative eigenvalue ($=-5.57$) is rather large.

Why would one even want to assume that dissimilarity data are Euclidean distances (except for an error component)? The justification must come from the way the data are generated or collected. If persons are asked directly for ratings on pairwise dissimilarities, then it may be plausible to hypothesize that the observed numerical responses are at least distance-like values. Such data could, therefore, be scaled directly using classical MDS. The procedure will show to what extent the data are indeed Euclidean distances.

Correlations as in Table 1.1, however, are definitely not Euclidean distances, but rather scalar products *by construction*. Thus, in this case, one should skip steps 1 and 2 in the above, and begin directly with step 3. This amounts to running a principal component analysis. An alternative approach is to first convert the scalar products to distances. In case of correlations, this conversion is $d_{ij} = \sqrt{2 - 2r_{ij}}$ (see formula 4.1 on page 46).

In case of larger errors (as in the example above), classical MDS quickly reaches its limits as a useful method. It generates a best-possible solution, but it does so minimizing a criterion known as *Strain* which is not as easily interpretable as Stress. Moreover, in most applications, the data are at best on an interval scale level. Hence, one would not want to interpret the data directly as distances, but rather allow for an optimal rescaling when mapping them into distances.

9.2 Iterative MDS Algorithms

Iterative MDS algorithms are more flexible than classical MDS. They find a Stress-optimal MDS configuration and, in doing so, they rescale the data optimally within the constraints of their scale level. However, iterative algorithms cannot guarantee to always find the global optimum solution, because their small-step improvements may

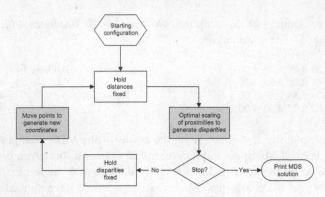

Fig. 9.1 Principles of an iterative MDS algorithm

get stuck in local minima. The user, therefore, should keep an eye on this possibility (see p. 77f. for suggestions on how to avoid local minimum solutions).

Iterative MDS algorithms proceed in two phases (see Fig. 9.1). In each phase one set of parameters (distances or disparities, respectively) is taken as fixed values, while the other set of arguments is modified in such a way that Stress is reduced:

1. The disparities (i.e., the admissibly transformed proximities) are fixed; the points in MDS space are moved (i.e., X_t is changed to become X_{t+1}) so that the distances of X_{t+1} minimize the Stress function.
2. The MDS configuration, X, is fixed; the disparities are rescaled within the bounds of their scale level so that the Stress function is minimized (*optimal scaling*).

If, after t phases, this ping-pong process does not reduce the Stress value by more than some fixed amount (e.g., 0.0005) or if the Stress value is even increasing, the search algorithm is stopped, and X_t is taken as the optimal solution.

Phase 1 amounts to a difficult mathematical problem with $n \cdot m$ unknown parameters, the values of X. To solve it, various optimization algorithms have been developed. The presently best algorithm is the SMACOF procedure (De Leeuw and Heiser 1980, Borg and Groenen 2005), because it guarantees that the iterations will converge to at least a *local* Stress minimum.[2] Other criteria can also be used to assess the quality of MDS algorithms (Basalaj 2001).

Phase 2 poses a relatively easy problem. In interval MDS, one solves the problem via linear regression. It finds the additive and multiplicative coefficients that linearly transform proximities into disparities such that the Stress is minimized for the given distances. For other MDS models, appropriate regression procedures are also available (e.g., monotone regression for ordinal MDS).

---

[2]SMACOF is an acronym for "Scaling by MAjorizing a COmplicated Function" (De Leeuw and Heiser 1980). The optimization method used by SMACOF is called "Majorization" (De Leeuw 1977, Groenen 1993). The basic idea of this method is that a complicated goal function (i.e., Stress within the MDS context) is approximated in each iteration by a less complicated function which is easier to optimize. For more details on how this method is used to solve MDS problems, see De Leeuw and Mair (2009) or Borg and Groenen (2005).

These issues are purely mathematical ones. Users of MDS need not be concerned with them. They should simply use MDS programs like drivers use their cars: Drivers have to know how to drive, but they do not have to understand the physics of combustion engines. Drivers, however, should also know how to run a car (e.g., making sure that it has enough gas), and MDS users must feed the programs properly and set the right options to get where they want to go, i.e., arriving at mathematically optimal and substantively meaningful solutions.

An important option is picking a good starting configuration. All MDS programs offer a few alternatives that users can try out to see if they all lead to the same solution. PROXSCAL, for example, allows its users to repeat the MDS process with many different *random* starting configurations, or pick a particular *rational* starting configuration (e.g., one that results from using classical MDS),[3] or use an *external* user-constructed starting configuration.

We recommend to always actively influence the choice of the starting configuration rather than leaving it to the MDS program to construct such a configuration internally. A good choice is often using a starting configuration constructed on substantive-theoretical grounds. One example is using the design configuration in Fig. 2.4 as a starting configuration when scaling the rectangle similarity data. If such an external configuration can be formulated, one should at least test it out in case the MDS program does not arrive at the expected solution with its internal options.

Depending on the particular MDS program, various "technical" options are always offered to MDS users. These options can strongly impact the final MDS solution, because they often prevent the algorithm from terminating its iterations even though the Stress can be further improved. In the GUI window of SYSTAT's MDS program shown in Fig. 1.5, for example, the user can set the maximum number of iterations and define a numerical criterion of convergence. For historical reasons (i.e., to save time and costs), the default values for these parameters are universally set much too defensively in all MDS programs so that the iterations are terminated too early. Users should set these parameters such that the program can do *as many iterations as necessary* to reduce Stress (see Sect. 7.2, p. 77). Computing time is not an issue with modern MDS programs.

9.3 Summary

If the data are Euclidean distances (apart from error), classical MDS is a convenient algebraic method to do MDS. It assumes that the dissimilarity data are Euclidean distances, converts them to scalar products, and then finds the MDS configuration by eigen-decomposition. Iterative algorithms are more flexible: They allow optimal rescalings of the data, and different varieties of Minkowski distances, not just Euclidean distances. Such programs begin by computing or using a starting con-

---

[3]Such options are sometimes called KRUSKAL, GUTTMAN, YOUNG or TORGERSON, depending on their respective inventors or authors (see also Fig. 1.5 and Fig. 10.4).

figuration, and then modify it by small point movements reducing its Stress. The distances of this configuration are then used as targets for optimally rescaling the data (thereby generating disparities) within the bounds of the data's scale level. This process of modifying the MDS configuration (with fixed disparities) and rescaling the disparities (with fixed distances) is repeated until it converges. The presently best algorithm for moving the points is SMACOF; rescaling the data is done by regression.

References

Basalaj, W. (2001). Proximity visualisation of abstract data, Unpublished doctoral dissertation, Cambridge University, U.K.

Borg, I., & Groenen, P. J. F. (2005). *Modern multidimensional scaling* (2nd ed.). New York: Springer.

De Leeuw, J. (1977). Applications of convex analysis to multidimensional scaling. In J. R. Barra, F. Brodeau, G. Romier, & B. van Cutsem (Eds.), *Recent developments in statistics* (pp. 133–145). Amsterdam: North Holland.

De Leeuw, J., & Mair, P. (2009). Multidimensional scaling using majorization: SMACOF in R. *Journal of Statistical Software*, *31*(3), 1-30. Retrieved from http://www.jstatsoft.org/v31/i03/.

De Leeuw, J., & Heiser, W. J. (1980). Multidimensional scaling with restrictions on the configuration. In P. R. Krishnaiah (Ed.), *Multivariate Analysis* (Vol. V, pp. 501–522). Amsterdam: North-Holland.

Groenen, P. J. F. (1993). The majorization approach to multidimensional scaling: some problems and extensions, Unpublished doctoral dissertation, University of Leiden.

Chapter 10
MDS Software

Abstract Two modern programs for MDS are described: PROXSCAL, an SPSS module, and SMACOF, an R package. Commands and/or GUI menus are presented and illustrated with practical applications.

Keywords PROXSCAL · PREFSCAL · SMACOF

In this chapter, we turn to software for MDS and unfolding. MDS programs are contained in all major statistics packages. In SPSS there are even two MDS modules, plus an unfolding program. No single MDS program is generally superior to all others, and none offers all MDS models discussed in this book. Most MDS programs allow the user to do both ordinal MDS and also interval MDS. Some can also handle the INDSCAL model or varieties of this model. Few offer confirmatory MDS that allows the user to impose additional restrictions onto the MDS solution. Only one, PERMAP, offers the possibility to directly interact with the program dynamically.

10.1 PROXSCAL

The MDS program that may be accessible to most users and that also offers many MDS models together with technically up-to-date solution algorithms is PROXSCAL. It is one of the two MDS modules in SPSS. PROXSCAL contains all of the popular models (ratio MDS, interval MDS, ordinal MDS; INDSCAL and related models; weights for each proximity; a variety of different starting configurations; numerous options for output, plots, and saving results), but also some forms of confirmatory MDS (using external scales, enforcing axial regions). However, all MDS models in PROXSCAL offer only Euclidean distances; no Shepard plots are generated (only related plots such as transformation plots); and unfolding is cumbersome to run.[1]

---

[1] For unfolding using SPSS, we recommend a specialized program, called PREFSCAL .

© The Author(s) 2018
I. Borg et al., *Applied Multidimensional Scaling and Unfolding*,
SpringerBriefs in Statistics, https://doi.org/10.1007/978-3-319-73471-2_10

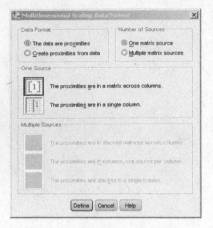

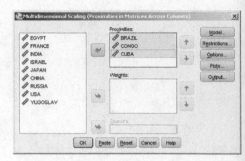

Fig. 10.1 Starting menu of PROXSCAL   **Fig. 10.2** Cardinal GUI menu of PROXSCAL

The user can interact with PROXSCAL via graphical menus or via commands. Menus are sufficient for most users. Moreover, they may be easier to use for beginners, and they print out the commands for later usage when applications need to be more fine-tuned and better documented.

The starting menu of PROXSCAL (in SPSS 19) is shown in Fig. 10.1 for the example discussed in Sect. 2.2. The program assumes that the user already imported the data into SPSS. This file is to be analyzed with MDS. Hence, no proximities have to be created by PROXSCAL. The user, therefore, checks the button in the upper left-hand corner, informing the program that the data are proximities.

If one begins with the usual "person × variable" data matrix of a social scientist, proximities must first be generated. PROXSCAL offers a few options for doing this if one checks the button "Create...". However, other modules in SPSS are usually better suited for computing proximities (e.g., inter-correlation routines). In this case, one first stores the proximities in some file, and then opens this file for MDS with PROXSCAL.

The remaining options in Fig. 10.1 are relevant only if one has more than just one data set, e.g., in case of INDSCAL modeling or if one has replicated proximities. If so, one can bind the k proximity matrices row-wise so that a $(k \cdot n) \times n$ matrix results. In order to keep track of the data, an additional variable is needed that denotes the different matrices. For example, this variable ("IDSource", say) may contain all 1's for the first matrix, then all 2's for the second, etc.

Figure 10.2 shows the main menu of PROXSCAL. In the upper right-hand corner, you find a set of buttons that call many options for running an MDS analysis of the given proximities. The most important ones are subsumed under the Model button. If you check this button, the menu in Fig. 10.3 appears.

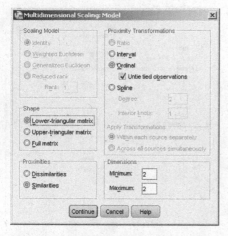

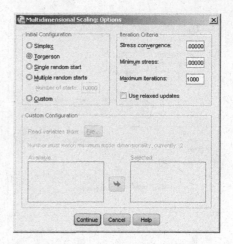

Fig. 10.3 Window with important model specification and data definitions

Fig. 10.4 Important nondefault specifications

For the country similarity data[2] used above in Sect. 2.2, we have to check in the lower left-hand corner of the menu in Fig. 10.3 that the data are Similarities. (The default setting is Dissimilarities. If you forget to set this properly, an MDS solution is computed that makes no sense and that has a very high Stress! Sometimes, one notices only then that something must have been misspecified.)

The menu, moreover, offers the user to specify the type of regression that the MDS program should use. For our example data, we specify that we want ordinal MDS, with the primary approach to ties ("untie").

Then, in the lower right-hand corner, we specify the dimensionality of the MDS solution(s). The default settings are "2", so there is just one two-dimensional solution. If you want higher dimensionalities as well, simply change Maximum to a higher value (e.g., 6). Note that unidimensional scaling solutions tend to have many local minima. Therefore, it is not recommended to set Maximum to 1 unless precautions are taken against local minima such as multiple random starts.

In the Shape box, we inform the program about the format of the proximity matrix. In publications, proximity matrices are often shown as lower-triangular matrices, and such data forms can be used as input too. There is no need to first assemble a full matrix.

The box in the upper left-hand corner of Fig. 10.3 is relevant only if you have more than 1 proximity matrix. If so, the option Weighted Euclidean yields an INDSCAL

---

[2]These data are available within SMACOF. You can export them from there into EXCEL, for example, by calling data(wish); M <- as.matrix(wish); require(foreign); write.xlsx(M, "WishData1.xlsx", row.names=FALSE) and then read the Excel file with SPSS.

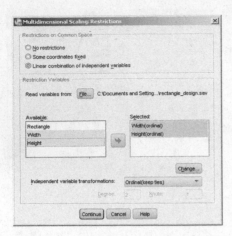 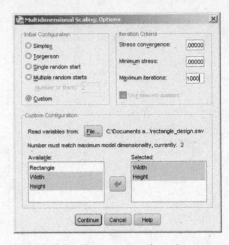

Fig. 10.5 External scales for confirmatory MDS

Fig. 10.6 Reading an external starting configuration into PROXSCAL

solution. In case of replicated data that are to be mapped into one distance each, you choose Identity.

Finally, the options of the PROXSCAL algorithm should be changed, because their defaults often lead to suboptimal MDS solutions. Fig. 10.4 shows how the options need to be set. First, change the initial configuration to Torgerson, that is, the classical scaling solution discussed in Sect. 9.1. Then, use stricter iteration criteria by setting Stress convergence and Minimum stress to 0.0000001 or smaller and Maximum iterations to at least 1000.

Leaving the rest of the buttons in this menu on their default settings, we can return to the cardinal menu in Fig. 10.2 via the "Continue" button. There, we click on "OK," and PROXSCAL will generate an MDS solution.

We now show how to formulate external restrictions on the dimensions of an MDS solution via the PROXSCAL menus. To demonstrate this, we use the rectangle data of Sect. 2.3. In the cardinal menu in Fig. 10.2, we click on Model Model to get to the menu that offers options on how the data should be transformed. In this menu (see Fig. 10.3), we inform the program that the data are dissimilarities; that they are stored in a lower triangular matrix; and that we want to run ordinal MDS with the primary approach to ties. Continue brings us back to the cardinal menu.

In the cardinal menu, we click on Restrictions. This brings us to the menu in Fig. 10.5. There, in the center of the window, we click on File and type the name of the SPSS file that contains the external scales into the space to the right of this button. Then, in the box on the left-hand side, we pick the variables that should serve as external scales, that is, "Width" and "Height." Finally, we request in the lower right-hand corner that these scales should be interpreted as ordinal scales and that the secondary approach to ties (keep ties) is to be used by the program.

We also want to use an external starting configuration for the MDS of the rectangle data. The window in Fig. 10.6 shows how to read this into PROXSCAL. We check Custom and write the name of the file with the external starting configuration into the window in the middle of the menu (here: "C:\Documents a..\rectangle_design.sav") that contains the coordinates of the design configuration of the rectangles. Its values are the physical coordinates of the rectangles used in the experiment. For the starting configuration, we select the variables "Width" and "Height" for the X- and Y-coordinates. With these specifications, the program yields a solution as in the right panel of Fig. 6.1.

10.2 The R Package SMACOF

R is a programming language as well as a statistical software environment.[3] R is available for free on CRAN (Comprehensive R Archive Network). The base package implements basic statistical and mathematical methods and functions. It can be extended by thousands of packages that offer additional methodologies.

To install the base distribution, the following steps need to be carried out:

- Go to http://CRAN.R-project.org
- Use the link "Download and Install R"
- Specify the operating system (OS) of your computer: R runs under MS Windows, Mac OS, and various Linux distributions
- Then, follow the remaining download instructions and install R

R provides efficient handling of vectors and matrices. A key feature of R is that outputs of statistical analyses are stored as R objects such as lists or matrices. The user can access these objects for further processing (very useful, in particular, for simulation studies). R also provides a powerful plot engine that allows for flexible customization of graphical output in publication quality. R is Open Source and issued under the GNU Public License (GPL), so the user has full access to the source code.

In order to work efficiently with R, an appropriate editor is required. We suggest using RSTUDIO; see http://rstudio.org and Verzani (2011).

There are several ways to import data into R. If the data are stored in EXCEL, SPSS, SYSTAT or similar formats, the foreign package can be considered which provides various utility functions. For EXCEL files in particular, it is suggested to save the spreadsheet as a csv file and then use the command read.csv() to import it into R. This function uses several default settings which the user may have to change depending on the Excel configuration. For instance, the following specification

```
read.csv(file, header=TRUE, sep=",", ...)
```

---

[3] As introductory books we suggest Venables and Smith (2002) (general introduction), Dalgaard (2008) and Everitt and Hothorn (2009) (introductory statistics with R).

implies that the first line contains the variable names and the variables are separated by a comma.

An SPSS file (here called XYZ.sav) can be imported directly using read.spss ("XYZ.sav") in the foreign package. If the file is not located in the R working directory, the user can specify a path such as read.spss("c:/data/XYZ.sav").[4]

10.2.1   Functions in SMACOF

The SMACOF package (De Leeuw and Mair, 2009) is available on CRAN. It implements a large variety of MDS models, many of them already covered in previous chapters. After launching RSTUDIO, the SMACOF package (as all other R packages as well) can be installed as follows:

```
R> install.packages("smacof")
```

The package installation needs to be done only once, unless you update the R version. Each time the R console is launched, the package needs to be loaded into working memory.

```
R> library("smacof")
```

At this point all functions and data implemented in smacof are available to the user. For a general package overview, the line

```
R> help(package="smacof")
```

opens the (HTML based) package documentation. The command

```
R> vignette("smacof")
```

opens the package vignette, a detailed description of the methodology including several examples.

The most important MDS functions implemented in smacof are the following:

- mds(): Simple MDS computation on a symmetric input dissimilarity matrix (see Chapters 1, 2, 3).
- indscal(), idioscal(): INDSCAL and IDIOSCAL models for individual differences MDS (see Chapter 5).
- smacofConstraint(): Confirmatory MDS with external constraints (see Chapter 6).

---

[4]For Windows user it is important to note that R always requires forward slashes when quoting a path.

- `smacofSphere()`: Spherical MDS (MDS with internal contraints: the points are restricted to be on a circle/sphere; see Chapter 6).
- `unfolding()`: Unfolding models (see Chapter 1 and 8).

Apart from the input dissimilarity matrix, the most important arguments in these functions are the following:

- ndim: number of dimensions of the MDS model (default: `ndim=2`).
- type: type of MDS model. The default is `type="ratio"`, other type options are `type="ordinal"`, `type="interval"`, and `type="mspline"`. For ordinal MDS, the default way of handling ties is `ties="primary"`, but it can be changed to `ties="secondary"`, or `ties="tertiary"`.
- init: initial configuration. For `mds()`, the default is `init="torgerson"`. It can be set to `init="random"` (in this case it is suggested to set a random number seed before the function call in order to get reproducible results), or a user-specified starting configuration matrix can be provided. Note that in case of unfolding, you have to specify a list with 2 initial configurations, one for the row points and one for the column points; see p. 97 for an example.

Other arguments can be found in the corresponding help files (by typing e.g. `?mds`).

Plotting is an important aspect in every MDS analysis. For each MDS model, SMA-COF provides numerous plotting options (see `?plot.smacof`. The most important plotting argument is `plot.type`. The default is `plot.type = "confplot"` which produces a configuration plot. For a Shepard plot the user needs to set `plot.type = "Shepard"`, for a bubble plot `plot.type = "bubbleplot"`, and for a Stress decomposition chart `plot.type = "stressplot"`.

In addition to the core MDS functions presented above, SMACOF provides numerous utility functions. One of these is `sim2diss()` which converts a similarity matrix to a dissimilarity matrix. This is important since all the MDS functions in SMACOF operate on input dissimilarities rather than input similarities. Details can be found in the corresponding help files.

For Stress evaluation the package implements `randomstress()` to simulate random Stress norms and `permtest()` to perform permutation tests (see Sects. 3.2 and 3.6). In order to examine the stability of a solution (see Sect. 3.7), `jackknife` and `bootmds()` can be used for MDS jackknife and bootstrap strategies, respectively. `Procrustes()` performs Procrustes transformations on two input configurations where one of the two acts as the target configuration (see Sect. 7.6). MDS biplots, where external variables are mapped into the configuration space, can be produced using `biplotmds()`.

The `icExplore()` function can be used to explore different random initial configurations as described in Sect. 7.3, and `stress0` (see Sect. 7.10) computes the Stress value for a zero-iteration MDS based on an initial configuration provided by the user.

Two more specialized models are asymmetric MDS (see Sect. 5.3) for which SMACOF implements the drift vector model by means of `driftVectors()`, and unidimensional scaling by means of the `uniscale()` function.

Finally, many datasets are included in the SMACOF package. They are used in this book (and in the package help files and the package vignette) to illustrate the various MDS models and SMACOF functions.

10.2.2   A Simple MDS Example

The R mantra is: "Everything in R is an object." Let us illustrate this concept (and some of the functionalities presented above) by means of a simple example. We use the Wish data, included in the package. They are provided as a similarity matrix. Therefore, the first step is to convert them to dissimilarities by subtracting each value from 7.[5]

```
R> wish.new <- sim2diss(wish, method=7)      ## convert similarities
R> wish.new                                  ## dissimilarities
         BRAZIL CONGO CUBA EGYPT FRANCE INDIA ISRAEL JAPAN CHINA RUSSIA  USA
CONGO      2.17
CUBA       1.72  2.44
EGYPT      3.56  2.00 1.83
FRANCE     2.28  3.00 2.89 2.22
INDIA      2.50  2.17 3.00 1.17  3.56
ISRAEL     3.17  3.67 3.39 2.33  3.00  2.89
JAPAN      3.50  3.61 4.06 3.17  2.78  2.50  2.17
CHINA      4.61  3.00 1.50 2.61  3.33  2.89  4.00  2.83
RUSSIA     3.94  3.61 1.56 2.61  1.94  2.50  2.83  2.39 1.28
USA        1.61  4.61 3.83 3.67  1.06  2.72  1.06  0.94 4.44  2.00
YUGOSLAV   3.83  3.50 1.89 2.72  2.28  3.00  2.56  2.72 1.94  0.33 3.44
```

This matrix of dissimilarities is assigned as an argument to the function mds()

```
R> res.wish <- mds(wish.new, type = "ordinal")  ## do MDS
```

The results are stored in the object res.wish. Some basic information can be accessed by just typing in the name of the object:

```
R> res.wish  ## basic output

Call:
mds(delta=wish.new, type="ordinal")

Model: Symmetric SMACOF
Number of objects: 12
Stress-1 value: 0.185
Number of iterations: 129
```

[5]Note that in this section the R> means that we are typing an individual command directly into the R console and then execute it by hitting the return key. Hence, you write a command, R responds, you then write the next command, R responds, etc. Normally, you would write a whole set of commands ("script") in the editor window, edit it, save it, and then "source" (i.e., execute) it.

All relevant SMACOF outputs are stored as single objects within the output list. The names of the list elements can be obtained by the names() command.

```
R> names(res.wish)
 [1] "delta" "dhat" "confdist" "iord" "conf" "stress" "spp" "ndim" "weightmat"
 "resmat" "rss"
 [2] "init" "model" "niter" "nobj" "type" "call"
```

The most important elements are:

- delta: Dissimilarity matrix.
- dhat: Optimally transformed dissimilarities (d-hats or disparities).
- confdist: Configuration distances computed from the MDS solution.
- conf: Configuration (coordinates) of the MDS solution ($\mathbf{X}$).
- stress: Stress-1 value.
- spp: Stress per point.
- niter: Number of iterations needed to fit the model.

As always in R, such list outputs can be accessed using the $ operator. For example, the matrix of the distances among the points of the MDS solution can be accessed using

```
R> res.wish$confdist
```

or, rounded to two decimal digits, by

```
R> round(res.wish$confdist, 2)
          BRAZIL CONGO CUBA EGYPT FRANCE INDIA ISRAEL JAPAN CHINA RUSSIA  USA
CONGO       0.74
CUBA        1.02  0.50
EGYPT       1.09  0.78 0.34
FRANCE      0.61  1.03 1.01  0.88
INDIA       0.81  0.73 0.49  0.32   0.56
ISRAEL      1.08  1.45 1.31  1.06   0.47  0.81
JAPAN       1.37  1.61 1.36  1.05   0.76  0.90   0.36
CHINA       1.65  1.32 0.82  0.57   1.32  0.84   1.33  1.15
RUSSIA      1.38  1.35 0.97  0.63   0.89  0.64   0.75  0.55  0.61
USA         0.97  1.47 1.42  1.23   0.44  0.94   0.29  0.64  1.57   1.02
YUGOSLAV    1.40  1.34 0.94  0.60   0.92  0.64   0.80  0.60  0.55   0.05 1.07
```

This distance matrix is an R object that can be used for further computations, or to produce plots.

A simple series of relevant plots can be produced as follows:

```
R> plot(res.wish)
R> plot(res.wish, plot.type = "Shepard")
R> plot(res.wish, plot.type = "bubbleplot")
R> plot(res.wish, plot.type = "stressplot")
```

Each of these plots can be customized using standard plotting arguments (and some more specialized ones). Examples are given in the plot.smacof help file.

References

Dalgaard, P. (2008). *Introductory statistics with R* (2nd ed.). New York: Springer.

De Leeuw, J., & Mair, P. (2009). Multidimensional scaling using majorization: SMACOF in R. Journal of Statistical Software , *31*(3), 1–30. Retrieved from http://www.jstatsoft.org/v31/i03/.

Everitt, B. S., & Hothorn, T. (2009). *A handbook of statistical analyses using R*. FL: Chapman and Hall.

Venables, W. N., & Smith, D. N. (2002). *An introduction to R*. Bristol: Network Theory Ltd.

Verzani, J. (2011). Getting started with RStudio: An integrated development environment for R. O'Reilly Media.

Index

A
Asymmetric data, 32, 57

B
Bootstrapping, 40

C
Circular MDS, 57, 72
Circular unfolding, 57
City-block distance, 16
Classical MDS, 81, 105
Cluster analysis, 91
Coarse data, 45
Confirmatory MDS, 67, 74
Convex hull, 22
Co-occurrence data, 47
Cylindrex, 20

D
Data
   automobiles, 68
   color similarity, 60
   countries, properties, 16
   countries, similarity, 14, 31, 79, 87
   crimes, frequencies, 1
   crimes, seriousness, 47
   dot patterns, 46
   employee survey, 11
   family conflicts, 48
   intelligence tests, 19
   journal references, 58
   KIPT, 82
   meaning of working, 47
   Morse signals, 58, 70
   occupational titles, 47
   organizational culture, 74
   personal values, 21, 22, 24, 73, 80
   rectangles, 18, 68, 80
   Republican voters, 50
   work values, 89
Degenerate solution, 81
Dimensional salience MDS, 60
Dimensional weighting MDS, 60, 68
Disparities, 30
Dominance metric, 16
Drift vector, 58
Drift vector model, 58

E
Euclidean distance, 16, 57, 109
Exploratory MDS, 67, 68, 74
External unfolding, 24, 95

F
Facet diagram, 89
Feature model distance, 46

G
Global minimum, 81
Gravity model, 49

I
icExplore, 88
IDIOSCAL, 62
Incidence matrix, 47, 50
Individual differences MDS, 60
INDSCAL, 60

© The Author(s) 2018
I. Borg et al., *Applied Multidimensional Scaling and Unfolding*,
SpringerBriefs in Statistics, https://doi.org/10.1007/978-3-319-73471-2

Initial configuration, 68, 78, 81, 109
Interval MDS, 30, 32, 54, 83
Iterations, 1, 108

L
Local minimum, 81

M
MDS algorithms, 72, 105
Metric MDS, 53
Missing data, 39, 44
Multi-start, 78

N
Non-metric MDS, 53

O
Ordinal MDS, 32, 53, 83

P
Permutation test, 35
Principal axis, 6, 86
Procrustes, 63, 79
Programs
    CMDA, 70
    EXCEL, 115
    PERMAP, 111
    PINDIS, 63
    PREFSCAL, 111
    PROXSCAL, 2, 78, 111
    R environment, 3, 115
    RSTUDIO, 4
    SMACOF package, 3, 115
    SPSS, 2, 112, 115
    SYSTAT, 3, 115

R
Radex, 20
Random data, 33, 39
Random Stress norms, 34
Ratio MDS, 30, 32, 55, 83
Raw Stress, 33
Regional interpretation, 89
Replicated data, 63
Representation errors, 31
R function
    boot(), 41
    CircE(), 74
    data(), 14
    driftVectors(), 59
    fitCircle(), 22, 24

hist(), 35
icExplore(), 79
idioscal(), 62
indscal(), 60
jackknife(), 39
lda(), 27
lm(), 27, 88
mds(), 8, 9, 22
permtest(), 35, 39
plot.Hulls(), 22
plot3d(), 96
Procrustes(), 84
random.multistart(), 78
randomstress(), 33
sim2diss(), 3, 32
smacofConstraint(), 68, 69
smacofIndDiff(), 60
smacofSphere(), 72
Stress0(), 79, 91
unfolding(), 10, 24
uniscale(), 81
vmu(), 102

S
S-coefficients, 48
Shepard diagram, 8, 29, 82, 83
Spherical MDS, 72
Spline transformation, 56
SPP, 36, 86
Starting configuration, 78, 109
Stress, 29, 85
Stress-1, 32, 33
Stress per Point, 36
Symmetric data, 32

T
Thurstone scaling, 47
Ties, primary approach, 39, 54, 92
Two-phase algorithm, 108

U
Unfolding, 8, 23
    circular, 103
    external, 24, 95
    model, 8
    multi-dimensional, 99
    multiple, 99
    vector model, 101
    weighted, 101

W
Weighted MDS, 64

Printed in the United States
By Bookmasters